INFECTIOUS DISEASES AND MICROBIOLOGY

IMPACTS AND IMPLICATIONS OF COVID-19

AN ANALYTICAL AND EMPIRICAL STUDY

Infectious Diseases and Microbiology

Additional books and e-books in this series can be found on Nova's website under the Series tab.

Infectious Diseases and Microbiology

Impacts and Implications of COVID-19

An Analytical and Empirical Study

Anand Sharma
Prateek Agrawal
Vishu Madaan
and
Anuj Agarwal
Editors

nova
Medicine & Health
New York

https://doi.org/10.52305/WZTU8416

Library of Congress Cataloging-in-Publication Data

ISBN: 978-1-53619-670-2

Published by Nova Science Publishers, Inc. † New York

CONTENTS

Preface

Coronaviruses (CoV) are a large family of viruses that cause illnesses ranging from the common cold to more severe diseases such as Middle East Respiratory Syndrome (MERS-CoV) and Severe Acute Respiratory Syndrome (SARS-CoV). Coronavirus disease (COVID-19) is a new strain that was emerged in Wuhan, China, in December 2019 and declared a pandemic by the World Health Organization (WHO) on March 11, 2020.

The outbreak of coronavirus disease 2019 (COVID-19) has created a global health crisis that has had a deep impact on the way we perceive our world and our everyday lives. COVID-19 is spreading across the world at an alarming speed. Not only the rate of contagion and patterns of transmission threatens our sense of agency, but the safety measures put in place to contain the spread of the virus also require social distancing by refraining from doing what is inherently human, which is to find solace in the company of others. Within this context of physical threat, social and physical distancing, as well as public alarm, what has been (and can be) the role of the different stakeholders in our lives on individual, social and societal levels?

This is an unprecedented crisis and calls for unprecedented measures. It is affecting human health, healthcare systems, global economy, business trades, manufacturing and service industries, transportation, etc. Nowadays, the government, policymakers, researchers, sociology professionals, medical as well as natural sciences have been working instantly to deal with, deriving solutions, spreading positivity, and trying to protect humankind against COVID-19; there is also a great focus on technological developments for improving the processes and mechanism for a better tomorrow.

The objective of the edited book is to provide the most recent research and innovative developments regarding the COVID-19. In this context, the book aims to inform the target audience about the latest findings-results regarding a wide variety of psychological, social, managerial, and technological issues for fighting COVID-19 and reform the world. The book is focused on the scientific research works targeting COVID-19 only. The emphasis is given on socio-economical, managerial, and alternative works giving insights about the impact of COVID-19.

Anand Sharma
Prateek Agrawal
Vishu Madaan
Anuj Agarwal

SECTION 1. DEALING WITH COVID-19

In: Impacts and Implications of COVID-19 ISBN: 978-1-53619-670-2
Editors: Anand Sharma et al.

Chapter 1

Machine Learning and AI Application of COVID-19 Pandemic Outbreak

***Ranjit Barua*[1,*], *Sudipto Datta*[1], *Pallab Dutta*[2] *and Amit Roy Chowdhury*[1,3]**

[1]Centre for Healthcare Science and Technology,
Indian Institute of Engineering Science and Technology, Shibpur,
Howrah, West Bengal, India
[2]National Institute of Pharmaceutical Education and Research
(NIPER) Kolkata. West Bengal, India
[3]Aerospace Engineering & Applied Mechanics,
Indian Institute of Engineering Science and Technology, Shibpur,
Howrah, West Bengal, India

Abstract

A novel coronavirus, also known as SARS-CoV-2, first spread in Wuhan city China in late 2019 from a seafood market and is spreading worldwide. WHO, i.e., World Health Organization, on January 30th, 2020, mentioned and declared this novel coronavirus outbreak as an emergency of public health at the international level. In the current situation, scientists, researchers, medical experts, and

* Corresponding Author's E-mail: ranjitjgec007@gmail.com.

clinicians find an alternative technology to handle the pandemic situation due to COVID-19. ML or Machine Learning had an essential impact on previous epidemic situations; therefore, the researchers are looking forward to overcoming the COVID-19 crisis. This chapter thoroughly discusses how the modern Machine Learning process involves the COVID-19 pandemic and helps fight against it. The constant growth in Machine Learning has a significant improvement in prediction, forecasting, screening, contact tracing, treatment, medication, and drug or vaccine invention process for COVID-19 and decreasing human interference in the healthcare system. The ongoing developments in Machine Learning have significantly improved treatment, medication, screening, prediction, forecasting, contact tracing, and drug/vaccine development process for the Covid-19 pandemic and reduce the human intervention in medical practice.

Keywords: COVID-19, outbreak, machine learning, SIR, SEIR, WHO

INTRODUCTION

By late 2019, a novel virus started spreading in Wuhan city of China from a Seafood market. This virus spread very fast from Wuhan to worldwide within a couple of months. It is soon identified that the virus belongs to a family of viruses known as coronaviruses like SARS and MERS having spikes on the outer surface of the spherical virus. Those spikes act as a key for specific human lung cells; by lock and key mechanism, the virus attaches with the human lung cells and infects the host. This new novel coronavirus was named SARS-CoV-2. It is very much similar to SARS-CoV because the new coronavirus also causes severe acute respiratory syndrome and high homology, i.e., 80% like SARS-CoV of 2003 [1]. The novel coronavirus was thought to have been transmitted from seafood animals like the zoonotic mode of transmission. Still, this assumption was proved wrong as later it was found out that human to the human model of communication also played a significant role in the subsequent outbreak [2]. WHO, i.e., World Health Organization, initially named the novel coronavirus as 2019-nCoV on January 12th, 2020. Later, WHO changed the name to 2019 coronavirus, i.e., COVID-19. Meanwhile, CSG (Coronavirus Study Group) of the international committee proposed to change the name from COVID-19 to SARS-CoV-2 issued on February 11th, 2020. Till January 14th, 2021 (11:49 am CET), 90,759,370 number of confirming COVID-19 cases are reported [3], whereas the maximum points have been noticed in the region of America (40,187,505), and the minimum instances have been seen in the Western Pacific region (1,227,622) [Figure 1].

On January 7th, 2020, the researchers of China isolated a SARS-CoV-2 virus from an infected patient and studied done genomic sequencing [1]. Soon WHO declared the new virus outbreak as a pandemic. SARS-CoV-2 infected approximately 200 countries worldwide [4, 5]. The present research suggests that Machine Learning is an advanced level technology hired by several medical organizations. Its outcome is more significant speed-up, scale-up handling power, consistent and also excel the human in a few particular medical practice [6]. Thus, medical organizations and healthcare practitioners worldwide are involved in several applications of the Machine Learning process to prevent the COVID-19 situation [7-9]. Present research emphasizes the outlook of Machine Learning for several pandemic occurrences (Figure 2); it helps medical specialists in numerous non-communicable diseases like heart disease, diabetes, cancer [10-12] and infectious diseases like COVID-19, HIV, EBOLA, etc. [13, 14].

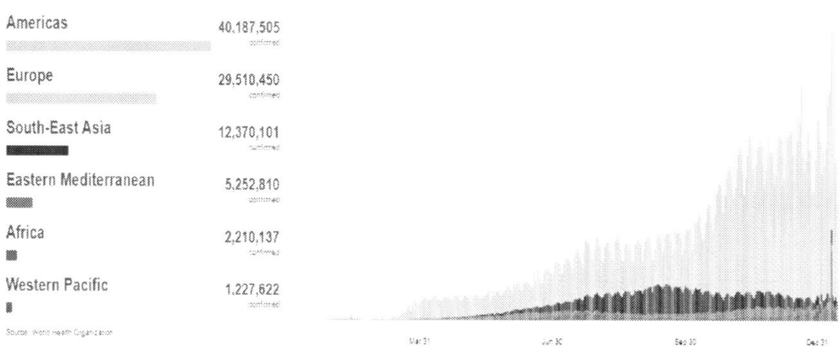

Figure 1. Active COVID-19 report by WHO [January 14th, 2021; 11:49 am CET].

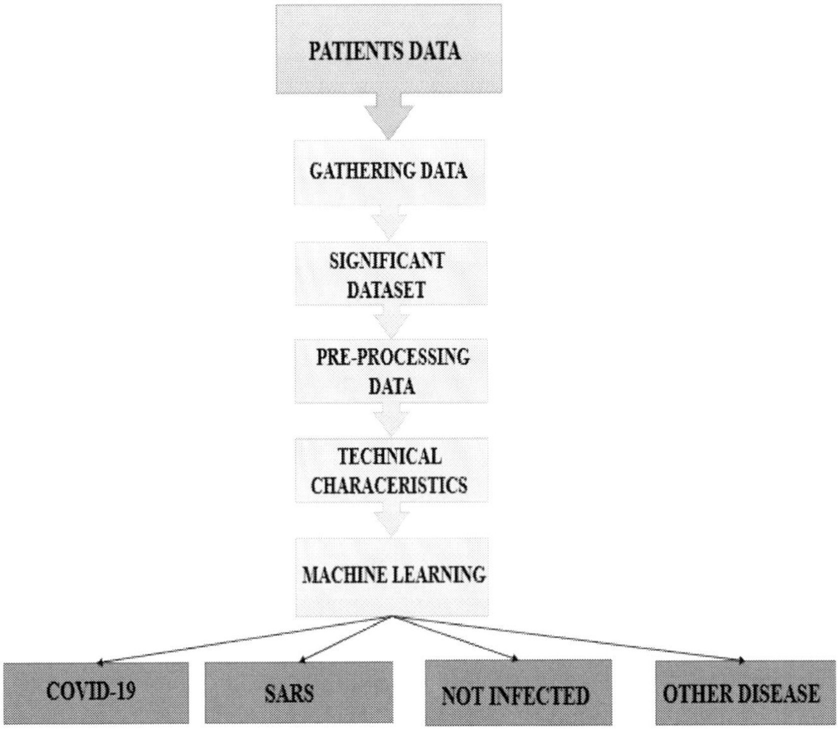

Figure 2. Machine Learning involves in the modern healthcare system.

Application of Machine Learning in COVID-19

Machine Learning has established excellent performance for various applications of image processing like image classification [15], image analysis [16, 17], also image segmentation [18]. Image classification was obtained by removing the significant characteristics from the descriptive images like image moment [19] or SIFT [20]. Afterward, these characteristics can be applied in the organizing task by organizers like SVM [21]. Some models like 'SIR,' 'SEIR,' are used in COVID-19 cases.

SIR Model

This model can demonstrate the change of infection rate with time (Figure. 3). If the number of individuals suspects is S_N, the number of individuals infectious is I_N, and the number of individuals recovered or deceased is R_N in any fixed area. Then,

$$\frac{dS_N}{dt} = -\frac{\beta I_N S_N}{N} \tag{1}$$

$$\frac{dI_N}{dt} = \frac{\beta I_N S_N}{N} - \gamma I_N \tag{2}$$

$$\frac{dR_N}{dt} = \gamma I_N \tag{3}$$

where β denotes the rate of contact in between the group of a suspect and infect; γ denotes the rate of transition in between the groups of infect and recovery.

If '$\Delta T'$' is the period of the pandemic situation within a particular area and at the same time the total population of this area $[n(\Delta T)]$ is assumed constant, then it can be written as:

$$n(\Delta T) = S_N + I_N + R_N = C \tag{4}$$

$\frac{dI_N}{dt} > 0,$ When the individual infected patients increase constantly, i.e.,

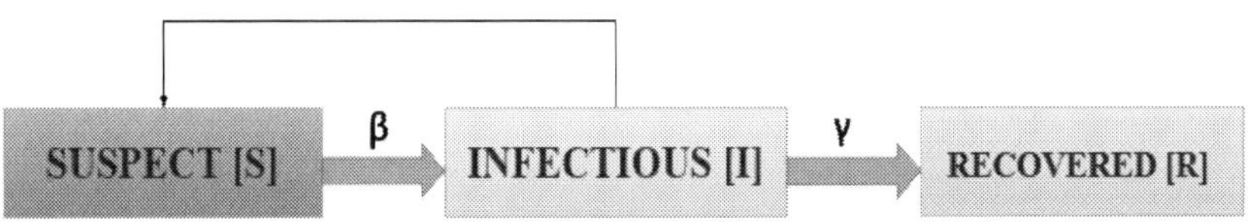

Figure 3. SIR model.

$$\frac{\beta}{\gamma} \times \frac{S_N}{N} > 1 \quad (5)$$

Where $\frac{\beta}{\gamma}$ is known as reproduction rate (R_r).

A SIR model [22] has been analyzed to predict the COVID-19 scenario in INDIA, shown in Figure 4, which shows the recorded data (confirm cases, recover cases, and fatality cases) COVID-19 in India from the beginning till April 2020.

SEIR Model

This model can demonstrate the incubation period of any epidemic disease (Figure 5). In this model, a new parameter is added, i.e., 'the number of exposed (E_N),' if the number of individuals suspect is S_N, the number of individuals infectious is I_N, and the number of individuals recovered or deceased is R_N in any fixed area. Then,

$$\frac{dS_N}{dt} = -\frac{\beta I_N S_N}{N} \quad (6)$$

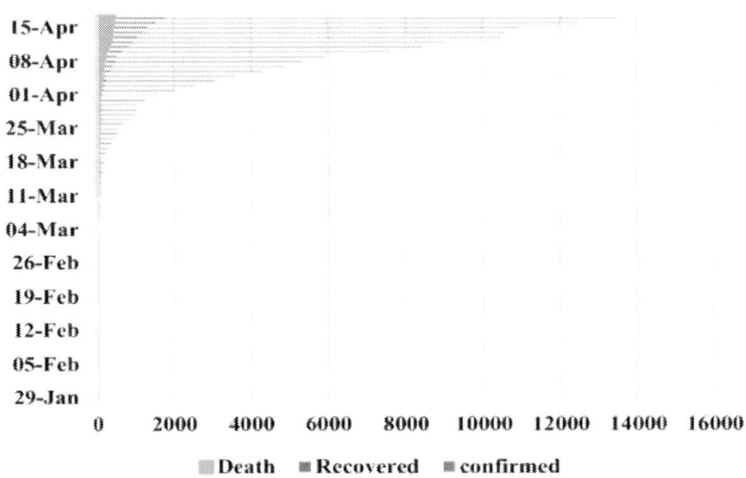

Figure 4. SIR model for predicting the COVID-19 cases in India [22].

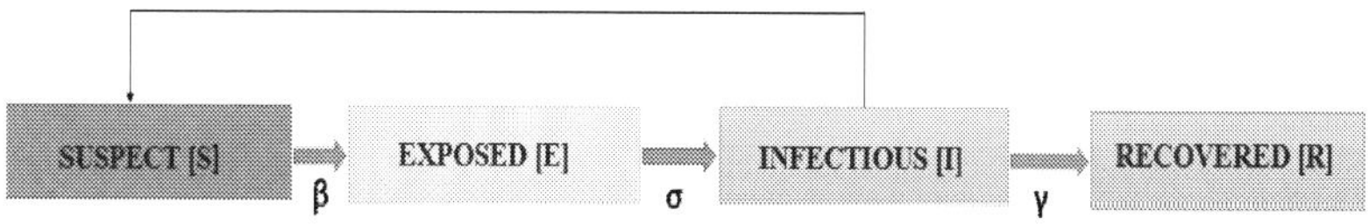

Figure 5. SEIR model.

$$\frac{dE_N}{dt} = \frac{\beta I_N S_N}{N} - \sigma E_N \tag{7}$$

$$\frac{dI_N}{dt} = \sigma E_N - \gamma I_N \tag{8}$$

$$\frac{dR_N}{dt} = \gamma I_N \tag{9}$$

Where β denotes the rate of contact between the group of a suspect and infect; γ indicates the rate of transition in between the groups of infect and recovery. If total population of any particular area $[n(\Delta T)]$, then;

$$n(\Delta T) = S_N + E_N + I_N + R_N \tag{10}$$

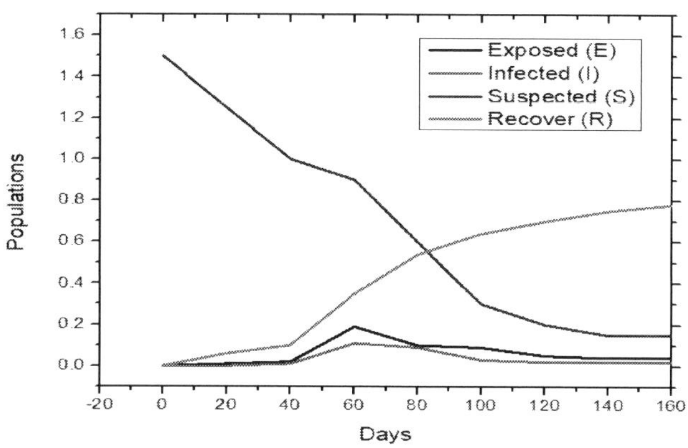

Figure 6. SEIR model analysis for a particular area of populations 965 million.

For instance, let us consider 965 million persons suspected of COVID-19, believe that only one person got infected in an initial phase, without any interference, the SEIR model for 160 days can be represented by Figure 6, where the suspected persons coincide with recovered patients at 80 days.

Compared to handmade characteristics, the deep neural networking technique [23] delivers excellent performance in sorting the images allowing the extracted structures. According to the Machine Learning features, numerous applications applied machine learning techniques to specify chest x-ray into standard cases and COVID-19 cases. Deep learning techniques use all these applications. For example, a CNN model was suggested from chest X-Ray images for the automatic diagnosis of COVID-19 [24]. With the help of Mobile-Net architecture, the accurate outcome is 96.78% [25]. Likewise, the conducted research used the transfer learning approach [26], and an accuracy rate is 97% was reported.

ML for Diagnosis and Screening

Identifying any disease (infectious and non-infectious) in the initial phase is really difficult but equally crucial to saving more lives [27, 28]. Rapid diagnosis and screening procedures can avoid the spread of pandemic situations like COVID-19, economical, and speedy recovery. Machine Learning is applied as a supplement in diagnosing and screening the recognized patient with radio imaging technology similar to X-Ray [7], CT scan (Computed Tomography), and Clinical blood sample data. In this concern, specific information on diagnosis and screening is suggested for the COVID-19 disease. The medical specialist can use radiology images like CT scans and X-rays as traditional methods to enhance conventional diagnosis and screening. Unluckily, the functioning of such devices is adequate during the crucial phase of the COVID-19 pandemic. In this respect, the researchers [29] indicate the prospect of Machine Learning technology by proposing the latest model, which gives a fast and effective COVID-19 diagnosis by the Deep Convolutional Network method.

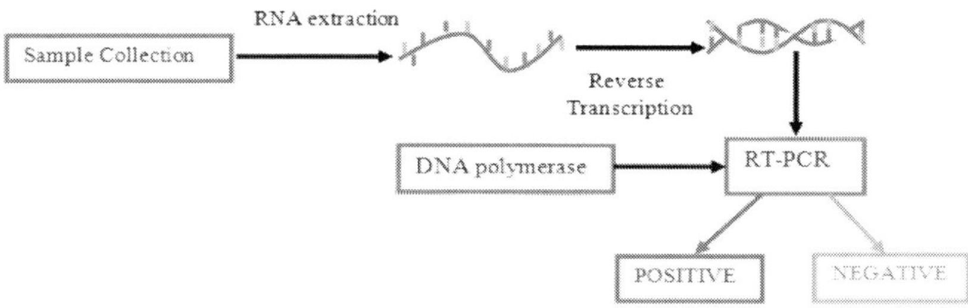

Figure 7. RT-PCR test procedures.

Table 1. Application of ML and AI in COVID-19 screening

Methods	No. of Patients	Data Types	Validation Procedure	Size of Samples	Accuracy
Support Vector Machine [33]	336, 220	Demographics Clinical, laboratory features,	Holdout	336 infected patients with PCR kit, 26 severe/critical cases, and 310 non-serious cases and with another related disease79 hypertension, 29diabetes, 17 coronary diseases, and 7 have a history of tuberculosis	Accuracy: 77.5% Specificity: 78.4% AUROC reaches 0.99 training and 0.98 testings dataset
CNN DarkCovidNet Architecture [34]	127, 43FM, 82 M 500, 500	Clinical, Mammographic	Cross-validation	127 X-ray images with 43 female and 82 male positive cases, 500 no-findings, and pneumonia cases of 500	Accuracy: 98.08% on Binary classes Accuracy: 87.02% on Multi-classes
Deep CNN ResNet-101 [26]	1020, 86	Clinical, Mammographic	Holdout	1020 CT images of 108 volume of patients with laboratory-confirmed Covid-19, 86 CT images of viral and atypical pneumonia patients,	Accuracy: 99.51% Specificity: 99.02%

The typical diagnostic method is the RT-PCR (Reverse Transcription-Polymerase Chain Reaction) method [30], a laboratory process that communicates with other RNA (Ribonucleic acid) and DNA (Deoxyribonucleic acid) to control the volume of exact RNA with the use of fluorescence (Figure 7). RT-PCR tests are done on clinical study tests of nasal secretions. The laboratory samples are taken by swab insertion into the nostril and softly moving it into the nasopharynx to gather secretions. Though RT-PCR can detect the coronavirus strain which causes COVID-19, in few test, it gave the result negative although the CT scan report of the patients showing improvement [31]. Numerous research [32-35] have claimed using X-rays and CT scans rather than RT-PCR due to its restricted accessibility in certain countries. Table 1 displays selective statistics on diagnosis and screening planned for the COVID-19 pandemic.

ML for Identification of COVID-19 Disease

When a person is detected with COVID-19, the following initial stage is most vital to stop the spread of COVID-19. As per WHO (World Health Organization), the virus spreads from person to person initially by droplets, saliva, or releases from the nose via contact transmission [38]. Contact tracing is an essential public medical care tool to control the COVID-19 transmission and to break the chain of virus transmission [39]. The procedure of contact tracing is to recognize and prevent the people who are recently coming in contact with an infected COVID-19 patient from stopping future transmission. Usually, the procedure acknowledges the infected patient with 14 days of quarantine. If this process is maintained, it can prevent the spread of the COVID-19 disease and decrease the pandemic outbreak. Several COVID-19 infected countries introduced many digital applications to trace the process with innovative applications and technologies like GPS (Global Positioning System), Bluetooth, Contact details, Social graph, Network-Based API, Card Transaction, System Physical Address, and Mobile Tracking Data. The symptoms of COVID-19 identified in the lower portion of the lungs have a higher precision when X-rays or CT scans are done than that when RT-PCR is conducted [40].

In some cases, RT-PCR tests can be replaced in place of X-ray or CT scans tests. Though, RT-PCR cannot identify the problem due to fewer radiologists than the populations. To control the issues of X-rays and CT scans and help radiologists, we have to recover the speed of the process. The purpose is to decrease the duration and work needed to execute X-rays and CT scans of COVID positive cases and calculate the amount of disease growth [41-43]. Radiological imaging is measured as an effective screening technique for the COVID-19 test [44]. It is observed that the features of COVID-19 are similar to pneumonia [28]. While performing a CT scan, all the COVID-19 patients were diagnosed with the same characteristics.

ML for Drugs and Vaccination

Due to the outburst of the Coronavirus pandemic, scientists and medical specialists worldwide universally advised to invent drugs and vaccines to prevent the COVID-19 pandemic, and the Machine Learning technique establishes to be a fascinating read. A new model is proposed to enhance the development of new drugs [45]. Two different datasets, i.e., one applying the 3C-like protease constraint and another data-holding record of infected COVID-19, HIV, influenza, etc. were used with the Machine Learning technique help of a deep neural networking process on 80 old drugs with possible treatment of COVID-19. The research recommended eight different drugs like Gemcitabine, Vismodegib, Celecoxib, Clofazimine, Conivaptan, Brequinar, Tolcapone, and Bedaquiline are shown practically effective against feline infectious peritonitis coronavirus. An antiviral drug is needed to handle the COVID-19 situation for which an innovative molecule modifier-drug target communication model was suggested [46].

A fusion of docking application with computational screening method and Machine Learning for selecting an additional medication to examine on COVID-19 was suggested [47]. Researchers mention the effective detection of the Zika virus [48], Ebola [49], and knowledge gain from experience can be used for the drug invention of COVID-19 and future pandemic situations. To calculate required affinity standards concerning commercially accessible antiviral drugs and target proteins on COVID-

19, researchers applied NLP-based molecule transformer-drug target interaction (MT-DTI). It managed to classify antiretroviral medication, which might be active in contrast to COVID-19 [50]. Correspondingly, applying a knowledge graph named BenevolentAI and an archive of designed medical evidence, ML (machine learning) discovered [51]. Artificial intelligence can help in medical conclusion making concerning patients with SARS-CoV-2, counting triage results for the ideal usage of restricted health care assets [52]. Artificial intelligence augmented system was applied for simple chest radiographs to record and calculate the pulmonary progress of SARS-CoV-2 surrounded by hospitalized peoples, which assisted in detecting patients that required serious care [48]. Figure 8 shows the importance of ML (machine learning) and AI for the COVID-19 pandemic. Initial credentials of at-risk problems could more monitor healthcare persons to previous interference, resulting in better-quality conclusions. For example, numerous clinical factors created an artificial intelligence framework that could forecast corrosion even at preliminary performance, with more accuracy associated with logistic deterioration [53].

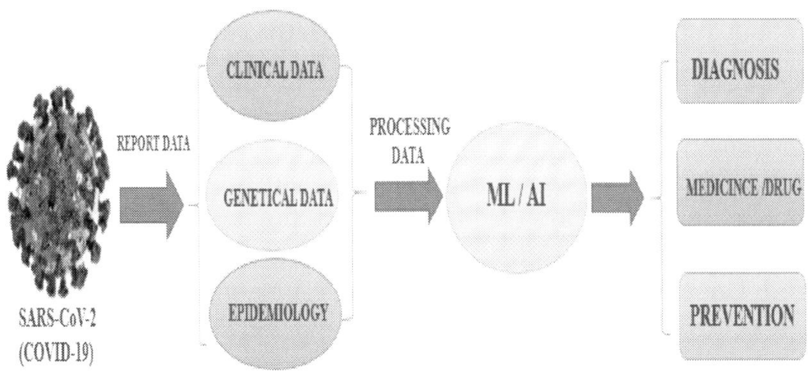

Figure 8. Application of ML/AI for COVID-19.

Conclusion

The constant progress in Machine Learning has a better impact on medication, treatment, screening, forecasting, prediction, contact tracing, and the improvement procedure of drugs and vaccine for the COVID-19, which decreases the social involvement in healthcare practice. SARS-CoV-2 is main responsible for the pandemic of COVID-19. It is imagined to belong to bat coronavirus and is also one of the seven human transmissible diseases. The first human case of coronavirus was noticed at Wuhan, China, in December of 2019. Those who have corona test positive are diagnosed as COVID-19 patients. Historical information and specific facts help make decisions using interacting technology like data mining and data analytics viewpoints. The size of the document accessible is vast and collecting facts and receiving the fascinating design out of the cumulated record is a difficult task. In this current emergency pandemic situation, Machine Learning plays an important role. This chance can later help in saving many lives, both in the present and in the future. Information and communication technology help in the decision-making process based on the past data with the data analytics and data mining perspective. The available data is vast; gathering information and getting an exciting pattern out of the cumulated data is challenging. Machine learning is a significant implement in fighting the present pandemic. If it was possible to take this prospect to collect data, pool the knowledge, and combine it with skills, it can save many lives – both now and in the future.

Acknowledgments

The authors would like to thank the Centre for Healthcare Science and Technology Lab, Heaton Hall, IIEST-Shibpur.

References

[1] Zhou, P; Yang, XL; Wang, XG; Hu, B; Zhang, L; Zhang, W; et al. A pneumonia outbreak associated with a new coronavirus of probable bat origin. *Nature.*, 2020. https://doi.org/10.1038/s41586-020-2012-7.

[2] Lu, R; Zhao, X; Li, J; Niu, P; Yang, B; Wu, H; et al. Genomic characterization and epidemiology of 2019 novel coronavirus:

implications for virus origins and receptor binding. *Lancet*., 2020, 395(10224), 565–74.

[3] WHO. *Coronavirus disease (COVID-2019) situation reports.* 2021. https://www.who.int/publications/m/item/weekly-epidemiological-update---12-january-2021.

[4] Barua, R; Datta, S; Roychowdhury, A; Datta, P. The Study of the Epidemiology and Clinical Features of the Novel Coronavirus (COVID-19), In S. Taukeni (Ed.), *Epidemiological Research Applications for Public Health Measurement and Intervention* (pp. 25-39). IGI Global.doi:10.4018/978-1-7998-4414-3.

[5] WHO. *Coronavirus disease (COVID-2019) situation reports.* 2020. https:// www.who.int/emergencies/diseases/novel-coronavirus-2019/situationreports. Accessed 5 Mar 2020.

[6] Sudipto Datta, Ranjit Barua, Jonali Das (December 12th 2019). *Application of Artificial Intelligence in Modern Healthcare System, Alginates - Recent Uses of This Natural Polymer*, Leonel Pereira, Intech Open, DOI: 10.5772/intechopen.90454.

[7] Akshat Agrawal, Rajesh Arora, Ranjna Arora, Prateek Agrawal. Applications of Artificial Intelligence and Internet of Things for Detection and Future Directions to Fight Against COVID-19. In an edited book on *Emerging Technologies for Battling Covid-19*, (2021), pp. 107-119, Springer.

[8] Madaan, V; Roy, A; Gupta, C; Agrawal, P; Sharma, A; Bologa, C; Prodan, R. *XCOVNet: Chest X-ray Image Classification for COVID-19 Early Detection Using Convolutional Neural Networks. New Generation Computing*, (2021), pp. 1-15, 2021. DOI: 10.1007/s00354-021-00121-7.

[9] Prateek Agrawal, Vishu Madaan, Aditya Roy, Rajani Kumari, Harshal Deore. FOCOMO: Forecasting and monitoring the worldwide spread of COVID-19 using machine learning methods, *Journal of Interdisciplinary Mathematics*, (2021), pp. 1-25. DOI: 10.1080/09720502.2021.1885812

[10] Saxena, S; Gyanchandani, M. Machine learning methods for computer-aided breast cancer diagnosis using histopathology: a narrative review, *J Med Imaging Radiat Sci*, (2019), 10.1016/j.jmir.2019.11.001.

[11] Kavakiotis, I; Tsave, O; Salifoglou, A; Maglaveras, N; Vlahavas, I; Chouvarda, I. *Machine learning and data mining methods in diabetes research Comput Struct Biotechnol J*, 15, (2017), pp. 104-116, 10.1016/j.csbj.2016.12.005.
[12] Liu, T; Fan, W; Wu, C. A hybrid machine learning approach to cerebral stroke prediction based on imbalanced medical dataset. *Artif Intell Med*, (2019), Article 101723, 10.1016/j.artmed. 2019.101723.
[13] Choi, S; Lee, J; Kang, MG; Min, H; Chang, YS; Yoon, S. *Large-scale machine learning of media outlets for understanding public reactions to nation-wide viral infection outbreaks Methods*, 129, (2017), pp. 50-59, 10.1016/j.ymeth.2017.07.027.
[14] Chockanathan, U; Dsouza, AM; Abidin, AZ; Schifitto, G; Wismüller, A. *Automated diagnosis of HIV-associated neurocognitive disorders using large-scale Granger causality analysis of resting-state functional MRI*, *Comput Biol Med*, 106, (2019), pp. 24-30, 10.1016/j.compbiomed.2019.01.006.
[15] Rawat, W; Wang, Z. "Deep convolutional neural networks for image classification: A comprehensive review;" *Neural computation*, vol. 29, pp. 2352–2449, 2017. pmid:28599112.
[16] Ke, Q; Zhang, J; Wei, W; Połap, D; Woźniak, M; Kośmider, L; et al., "A neuro-heuristic approach for recognition of lung diseases from X-ray images;" *Expert Systems with Applications*, vol. 126, pp. 218–232, 2019.
[17] Chouhan, V; Singh, SK; Khamparia, A; Gupta, D; Tiwari, P; Moreira, C; et al., "A Novel Transfer Learning-Based Approach for Pneumonia Detection in Chest X-ray Images;" *Applied Sciences*, vol. 10, p. 559, 2020.
[18] Yang, L; Zhang, Y; Chen, J; Zhang, S; Chen, DZ. "Suggestive annotation: A deep active learning framework for biomedical image segmentation," in *International conference on medical image computing and computer-assisted intervention*, 2017, pp. 399–407.
[19] Yang, Y; Newsam, S. "Comparing SIFT descriptors and Gabor texture features for classification of remotely sensed imagery," in *2008 15th IEEE international conference on image processing*, 2008, pp. 1852–1855.

[20] Elaziz, MA; Hosny, KM; Selim, I. "Galaxies image classification using artificial bee colony based on orthogonal Gegenbauer moments," *Soft Computing*, vol. 23, pp. 9573–9583, 2019.
[21] Suykens, JA; Vandewalle, J. "Least squares support vector machine classifiers," *Neural processing letters*, vol. 9, pp. 293–300, 1999.
[22] Venkatasen, M; Mathivanan, SK; Jayagopal, P; et al. Forecasting of the SARS-CoV-2 epidemic in India using SIR model, flatten curve and herd immunity. *J Ambient Intell Human Comput*, (2020). https://doi.org/10.1007/s12652-020-02641-4.
[23] Simonyan, K; Zisserman, A. "Intense convolutional networks for large-scale image recognition," *arXiv preprint ar X iv*:1409.1556, 2014.
[24] Apostolopoulos, ID; Mpesiana, TA. "Covid-19: automatic detection from x-ray images utilizing transfer learning with convolutional neural networks," *Physical and Engineering Sciences in Medicine*, p. 1, 2020.
[25] Narin, A; Kaya, C; Pamuk, Z. "Automatic detection of coronavirus disease (COVID-19) using X-ray images and deep convolutional neural networks," *arXiv preprint ar X iv*, 2003, 10849, 2020.
[26] Hosny, KM; Hamza, HM; Lashin, NA. "Copy-for-duplication forgery detection in color images using QPCETMs and sub-image approach," *IET Image Processing*, vol. 13, pp. 1437–1446, 2019.
[27] Vaishya, R; Javaid, M; Khan, IH; Haleem, A. *Artificial Intelligence (AI) applications for COVID-19 pandemic Diabetes Metab Syndr*, 14 (4), (2020), pp. 337-339, 10.1016/j.dsx.2020.04.012.
[28] Ai, T; Yang, Z; Hou, H; Zhan, C; Chen, C; Lv, W; Tao, Q; Sun, ZL. XiaCorrelation of chest CT and RT-PCR testing in coronavirus disease 2019 (COVID-19) in China: a report of 1014 cases. *Radiology*, (2020), https://doi.org/10.1148/radiol.2020200642.
[29] Ardakani, AA; Kanafi, AR; Acharya, UR; Khadem, N; Mohammadi, A. Application of deep learning technique to manage COVID-19 in routine clinical practice using CT images: results of 10 convolutional neural networks. *Comput Biol Med.*, 2020, 121 doi: 10.1016/j.compbiomed.2020.103795. 2020.
[30] World Health Organization, *Laboratory testing for coronavirus disease 2019 (COVID-19) in suspected human cases: interim*

guidance, 2 March 2020, World Health Organization, World Health Organization, 2020.

[31] Jiang, F; Deng, L; Zhang, L; Cai, Y; Cheung, CW; Xia, Z. "Review of the clinical characteristics of coronavirus disease 2019 (COVID-19)," *Journal of General Internal Medicine*, pp. 1-5, 2020.

[32] Wu, Z; McGoogan, JM. "Characteristics of and important lessons from the coronavirus disease 2019 (COVID-19) outbreak in China, summary of a report of 72 314 cases from the Chinese Center for Disease Control and Prevention," *Jama*, 2020.

[33] Maghdid, HS; Asaad, AT; Ghafoor, KZ; Sadiq, AS; Khan, MK. "Diagnosing COVID-19 Pneumonia from X-Ray and CT Images using Deep Learning and Transfer Learning Algorithms," *arXiv preprint arXiv*, 2004, 00038, 2020.

[34] Santosh, K. "AI-Driven Tools for Coronavirus Outbreak: Need of Active Learning and Cross-Population Train/Test Models on Multitudinal/Multimodal Data," *Journal of Medical Systems*, vol. 44, pp. 1-5, 2020.

[35] Wynants, L; Van Calster, B; Bonten, MM; Collins, GS; Debray, TP; De Vos, M; et al., "Systematic review and critical appraisal of prediction models for diagnosis and prognosis of COVID-19 infection," *medRxiv*, 2020.

[36] Sun, L; Liu, G; Song, F; Shi, N; Liu, F; Li, S; Li, P; Zhang, W; Jiang, X; Zhang, Y; Sun, L; Chen, X; Shi, Y. Combination of four clinical indicators predicts the severe/critical symptom of patients infected COVID-19. *J Clin Virol.*, 2020, doi: 10.1016/j.jcv.2020.104431.

[37] Ozturk, T; Talo, M; Yildirim, EA; Baloglu, UB; Yildirim, O; Rajendra Acharya, U. Automated detection of COVID-19 cases using deep neural networks with X-ray images. *Comput Biol Med.*, 2020 doi: 10.1016/j.compbiomed.2020.103792.

[38] WHO: World Health Organization, 2020. *Health Topic, Coronavirus disease overview.* https://www.who.int/health-topics/coronavirus#tab=tab_1(accessed May 29th, 2020).

[39] WHO: World Health Organization, 2020. *Contact tracing in the context of COVID-19.* (Accessed May 29th 2020). https://www.who.int/publications-detail/contact-tracing-in-the-context-of-covid-19.

[40] WHO: World Health Organization, 2020. *Contact tracing in the context of COVID-19.* (Accessed May 29th 2020). https://www.who.int/publications-detail/contact-tracing-in-the-context-of-covid-19.

[41] Mesleh, A. *Support Vector Machine Text Classifier for Arabic Articles*, ed: VDM Verlag Dr. Müller, 2010.

[42] Bukhari, SUK; Bukhari, SSK; Syed, A. SSH. SHAH, "The diagnostic evaluation of Convolutional Neural Network (CNN) for the assessment of chest X-ray of patients infected with COVID-19," *medRxiv*, 2020.

[43] Shi, H; Han, X; Jiang, N; Cao, Y; Alwalid, O; Gu, J; et al., "Radiological findings from 81 patients with COVID-19 pneumonia in Wuhan, China" a descriptive study," *The Lancet Infectious Diseases*, 2020.

[44] Feng, C; Elazab, A; Yang, P; Wang, T; Zhou, F; Hu, H; et al., "Deep Learning Framework for Alzheimer's Disease Diagnosis via 3D-CNN and FSBi-LSTM," *IEEE Access*, vol. 7, pp. 63605-63618, 2019.

[45] Ogunleye, AA; Qing-Guo, W. *"XGBoost model for chronic kidney disease diagnosis," IEEE/ACM transactions on computational biology and bioinformatics*, 2019.

[46] Ke, YY; Peng, TT; Yeh, TK; Huang, WZ; Chang, SE; Wu, SH; Hung, HC; Hsu, TA; Lee, SJ; Song, JS; Lin, WH; Chiang, TJ; Lin, JH; Sytwu, HK; Chen, CT. *Artificial intelligence approach fighting COVID-19 with repurposing drugs Biomed J*, (2020), 10.1016/j.bj.2020.05.001.

[47] Beck, BR; Shin, B; Choi, Y; Park, S; Kang, K. *Predicting commercially available antiviral drugs that may act on the novel coronavirus (SARS-CoV-2) through a drug-target interaction deep learning model Comput Struct Biotechnol J*, 18, (2020), pp. 784-790, 10.1016/j.csbj.2020.03.025.

[48] Ekins, S; Freundlich, J; Coffee, M. *A common feature pharmacophore for FDA-approved drugs inhibiting the Ebola virus F1000Research*, 3, (2014), p. 277.

[49] Ekins, S; Mottin, M; Ramos, PRPS; Sousa, BKP; Neves, BJ; Foil, DH; Zorn, KM; Braga, RC; Coffee, M; Southan, C; Puhl, CACH.

Andrade Déjà vu: stimulating open drug discovery for SARS-CoV-2 Drug Discov Today, (2020), 10.1016/j.drudis.2020.03.019.

[50] Ekins, S; Mietchen, D; Coffee, M; Stratton, TP; Freundlich, JS; Freitas-Junior, L; Muratov, E; Siqueira-Neto, J; Williams, AJ; Andrade, C. *Open drug discovery for the Zika virus*. F1000 Research., (2016).

[51] Beck, BR; Shin, B; Choi, Y; Park, S; Kang, K. Predicting commercially available antiviral drugs that may act on the novel coronavirus (SARS-CoV-2) through a drug-target interaction deep learning model. *Comput Struct Biotechnol J.*, 2020, 18, 784–790. doi: 10.1016/j.csbj.2020.03.025.

[52] Richardson, P; Griffin, I; Tucker, C; Smith, D; Oechsle, O; Phelan, A; Rawling, M; Savory, E; Stebbing, J. Baricitinib as potential treatment for 2019-nCoV acute respiratory disease. *The Lancet.*, 2020 Feb, 395(10223), e30–e31. doi: 10.1016/s0140-6736(20)30304-4.

[53] Jiang, X; Coffee, M; Bari, A. *Towards an Artificial Intelligence Framework for Data-Driven Prediction of Coronavirus Clinical Severity.*, 2020, March 30th, 63(1), 537–551. doi: 10.32604/cmc.2020.010691.

[54] Hurt, B; Kligerman, S; Hsiao, A. Deep Learning Localization of Pneumonia: 2019 Coronavirus (COVID-19) Outbreak. *J Thorac Imaging.*, 2020 May, 35(3), W87–W89. doi: 10.1097/RTI.0000000000000512.

[55] Paraskevis, D; Kostaki, EG; Magiorkinis, G; Panayiotakopoulos, G; Sourvinos, G; Tsiodras, S. Full-genome evolutionary analysis of the novel corona virus (2019-nCoV) rejects the hypothesis of emergence as a result of a recent recombination event. *Infect Genet Evol.*, 2020, 79, 104212.

[56] Dong, Y; Mo, X; Hu, Y; Qi, X; Jiang, F; Jiang, Z; Tong, S. *Epidemiological characteristics of 2143 Pediatric patients with 2019 coronavirus disease in China*, *Journal.*, (2020), https://doi.org/10.1542/peds.2020-0702.

[57] Giovanetti, M; Benvenuto, D; Angeletti, S; Ciccozzi, M. The first two cases of 2019-nCoV in Italy: where they come from? *J Med Virol.*, 2020, 1–4. https://doi.org/10.1002/jmv.25699.

Appendix A. Additional Information

COVID-19 disease caused by Novel Coronavirus, which is also known as SARS-CoV-2 or Severe Acute Respiratory Syndrome Coronavirus 2 [54], has converted an unmatched global health disaster. In December 2019, COVID-19 disease was noticed in Wuhan, China, and rapidly spread worldwide [55]. Many research works presented that the novel coronavirus or SARS-CoV-2 virus is mainly transmitted from bat to human inhabitants [56], and it is recommended that further spread of the COVID-19 epidemic was supported by human mobility and that quarantine of diagnosed or suspected cases is beneficial to avoid more transmission [57]. Globally 90,759,370 number of confirming COVID-19 cases have been reported to date (the maximum 40,187,505 confirmed cases has been noticed in the region of America, and the minimum 1,227,622 number confirmed cases had been noticed in the Western Pacific region) [3]. Presently lots of research work is going on the COVID-19 vaccine. With the help of modern technology like ML/AI, the data of the infected patients are analyzed to find the epidemiology, etiology and impact of COVID-19.

Appendix B. Key Terms and Definitions

COVID-19

A virus-infected disease caused by novel coronavirus or SARS-CoV-2, any persons, can be affected by other conduct like infected areas or droplets of any infected persons' cough or sneeze, or any bodily contact infected patients, etc. In December 2019, COVID-19 disease came in noticed in Wuhan, China.

Out-Breaks

An unexpected intensification in happenings of infection in any region during a specific period.

An unwelcome event like war or any virus transmission disease, etc.

Machine Learning

Machine learning the analysis of computer algorithms that recover automatically by practice. It is also known as an application of AI.

SIR

A SIR model is a mathematical model which calculates the hypothetical number of any disease-infected persons with a contagious infection in particular inhabitants over time.

SEIR

A mathematical model to establish the incubation period for any widespread disease.

WHO

A subsidiary body of the United Nations which basically in charge of the public health issues worldwide. The full name of WHO is “The World Health Organization”.

In: Impacts and Implications of COVID-19 ISBN: 978-1-53619-670-2
Editors: Anand Sharma et al.

Chapter 2

COVID-19: Clinical Management with Immunomodulator Therapy

Amit Kumar Verma[1,*], Preeti Mishra[2] and Vikas Saxena[3]

[1]Department of Pharmacy MJP Rohilkhand University Bareilly UP, India
[2]Raja Balwant Singh Engineering Technical Campus Bichpuri Agra UP, India
[3]Rakshpal Bhadur College of Pharmacy, Bareilly UP, India

Abstract

Cumulatively, nearly a Hundred million COVID-19 cases and twenty-three lakhs deaths were reported till 12 February 2021. The number of deaths was so reduced when compared with the previous week on 24-30 August. COVID-19 is an academic degree acute unwellness caused by SARS-CoV-2, mainly known to attack the lungs. Most COVID-19 patients experience fever, cough, fatigue, anorexia, and shortness of breath. There is an academic degree imperative need for effective interventions presently. Activity an irregular controlled trial with a placebo arm throughout a fatal death

* Corresponding Author's E-mail: professoramitmjpuniversity@gmail.com.

pandemic is very troublesome. Until herd immunity develops against SARS-CoV-2, ideally through effective vaccines, the worldwide population will keep in peril. The chapter deals with immunomodulatory therapy for the clinical management of patients.

Keywords: COVID-19, immunomodulator, Tulsi, Giloy, garlic

INTRODUCTION

Cumulatively, nearly twenty-seven million COVID-19 cases and 900000 deaths area unit consistent with United Nations agency to this purpose. As per the reports, COVID-19 new cases were almost 1.8 million with an estimated death of 37000 as of 6 September 2020. The number of deaths was so reduced when compared with the previous week on 24-30 August.

The United Nations Agency South-East Asia Region continued to purpose the most effective expansion thoroughly in new COVID-19 cases in the past week, in contrast to the previous week, with over 600000 new cases accordingly.

In Japan, Europe, and the Mediterranean regions, a rapid increase in COVID-19 cases was noticed that left all to worry. Opposite to this, the region of America and Western Pacific regions marked a decline in the new cases and death rate when compared [1]. Many types of research are taken place to predict the virus impact and detection [2-4].

The Region of America has seen the tenth increase in according cases, but a forty-five downfall in deaths, and continues to carry ultimately the most effective load of the unhealthiness globally.

COVID-19 is an academic degree acute unwellness caused by SARS-CoV-2 that affects the lungs and is claimed to mental, diarrhea, inflammatory disease, nausea, etc. [5]. Transmission of the SARS-CoV-2 virus can occur through various means that can be direct or indirect, which includes spitting, coming in contact with infected droplets, and secretions expelled out from the infected person, and medicine manifestations, amongst others. Most COVID-19 patients encounter the occurrence of fever, cough, fatigue, anorexia, and dyspnea. However, some other symptoms that were shown only in a few people are nasal congestion, headache.

The people infected with the coronavirus will experience different symptoms depending on their age, immunity-like factors. COVID-19 virus proved to be most dangerous for especially old age people suffering from former diseases like diabetes, chronic unwellness, and cancer.

The best way of preventing and hamper transmission is to search out about the COVID-19 virus, the problem this virus causes the way of its spreading and avoid all the necessary stuff that can increase the chance to get infected like not touching the face, proper cleaning of hands from time to time, rubbing of alcohol-based sanitizers, use of alcohol swabs to disinfect the gadgets, etc.

The COVID-19 virus spreads through various means, but most often, it can transmit the spitting or discharge of cough, sneezing of the already infected person that can only be prevented by following the instructions and guidelines like the use of a face mask, by coughing into a flexed elbow.

At now, there are not any particular vaccines or therapy for COVID-19, but still, many current clinical trials area unit evaluating and finding out the suitable treatments [6]. United Nations agency will still provide updated knowledge as presently as clinical findings become available.

There are mainly two types of defense systems: immunity, which works when an organism enters into the body.

Resistance Immunity

Resistance immunity involves various soluble and cell-based antimicrobial factors and works when infection occurs.

Adaptational Immunity

Adaptational immunity consists of pathogen-specific macromolecules and T-cells that develop immunity once they get infected and recover from it. The system is classically divided into innate and adaptational components [7]. The innate system provides non-specific resistance to pathogens, whereas adaptational immunity is characterized by substance and medical science memory specificity. Immunomodulators area unit drugs are that either restore or subdue the system.

The 2-immune systems, immunomodulators, work to avert and manage the infection. The COVID-19 pandemic represents one of the foremost widespread infectious challenges in recent times. COVID-19 is responsible for larger than 250,000 deaths worldwide and continues to increase daily [8]. COVID-19 is an academic degree acute unwellness caused by SARS-CoV-2. The design for effective anti-viral therapies and treatment is current. Immunogenic development is progressing quickly, but widespread immunogenic convenience is countable to be a minimum of 1 year away [9]. There is an academic degree imperative need for effective interventions presently. Activity an irregular controlled trial with a placebo arm throughout a deadly pandemic is very troublesome. Until herd immunity develops against SARS-CoV-2, ideally through effective vaccines, the worldwide population will keep in peril.

IMMUNOMODULATORS

Anti-Cytokines

The SARS-CoV-2-induced disease occurs by hyperactivation of effector T-cell and increased production of inflammatory cytokines, mainly IL-6. This reaction leads to having certain complications for the patient to take any type of antibodies, immunity based medical care, etc. This is called the macromolecule storm. IL-6, totally different cytokines (i.e., IL-1, TNF, and interferon-γ), that area unit created throughout the macromolecule storm, contribute to the process that takes it in plasma run, tube consistency, and disseminated intravascular curdling11. Due to all these problems, a rapid increase in the spreading of the virus was noticed. Tocilizumab was of little use for the treatment of patients as it was known to block IL-6 cytokine. It was also clear that medical care was enough to prevent and treat SARS-CoV-2 iatrogenic disease.

Most proteins are discharged throughout a protein storm and in the COVID-19 area unit created in high amounts throughout exacerbations of immune-mediated disorders and shows various therapeutic targets.

We tend to suppress the production of IL-6 by ingestion of IL-6 inhibitors can is somehow able to prevent the spread of SARS-CoV-2.

Though we tend to predict direct data in support of this hypothesis, doctors' and clinicians' advice was supposed to take macromolecule blockers and stay on medication till needed [10]. Along with all this, the best way found was to stay away from the infected patients and the places which have the higher chances to have COVID-19 infection and practice social distancing and self-quarantine.

Granulocyte- Scavenger Cell Colony

COVID-19 has involved the symptoms from very mild to even very severely that ultimately leads to the failure of the biological system of the human body, takes the patient on ventilation, and finally to death [11]. Many of the injuries were because of the outpouring of the inflammatory cytokines [interleukin-6, interferon-γ, and granulocyte-monocyte stimulating issue (GM-CSF)). Blunting this hyper inflammation with immunomodulation may cause clinical improvement. GM-CSF is created by many cells, likewise as macrophages and T-cells. Like alveolar macrophages (A.M.s), the GM-CSF is involved in the differentiation of macrophages. In animals, when their biological system gets infected, the administration of GM-CSF through intranasal route increase the rapid growth of A.M.s and gave improved result. Increased levels of GM-CSF area unit recently delineate in people suffering from COVID-19 compared to healthy controls [12]. GM-CSF has also been noticed to be helpful in the appropriate response; throughout this case, the inflammatory response is not enormously adaptive and not in the proportionate method.

In the severe cases of COVID-19 with people suffering from former diseases, the inhibition of the GM-CSF may come out to be helpful in the hyper inflammation-related injuries. The blockage of GM-CSF can be done by using antagonism of it or by the direct binding of GM-CSF. Initially, patients were treated with the macromolecule binding of GM-CSF receptor α called "Mavirilimumab," which showed impressive results by shortening the duration of hospitalization of patients. The clinical trial of patients is going to conduct the test of GM-CSF antibodies

TJ003234 and gimsilumab. Along with this, a drug named Lenzilumab has received approval from a federal agency for its use. These trials will facilitate inform whether or not or not blunting the inflammatory sign provided by the GM-CSF axis in COVID-19 is beneficial [13].

Convalescent Plasma

The convalescent plasma technique has no authorized vaccines at present for COVID-19 treatment. People who have recovered from COVID-19 contain the anti-SARS CoV-2 antibody plasma collected from them and administered to the patients suffering from the virus. The results seem to be in favor as they helped slow down the other treatments' requirements. It is known to be plasma therapy [14]. Due to this, C.P. came out to be known for the treatment of anti-viral medical care. 200-600 ml of plasma collected from the recovered patient with the suitable devices. C.P. was generally used for very critical patients because of the virus and was on the ventilator. The outcome was so secure and required no doubt and came out to be an effective treatment for COVID-19. It would even be used for prophylactic functions, but this approach's protection and effectiveness got to be tested in irregular prospective clinical trials.

The mechanism that how the C.P. is working was not known much, but some of the sources showed that the mechanism was the neutralization of antibodies, just like in the Ebola virus. It includes cellular toxicity, complement activation, and the body process. When CP is administered in the body, it provides management of the agent load. . Nonneutralizing antibodies may also contribute to the bar and/or enhance recovery [15].

Corticosteroids

Various serious injuries occurred due to a rapid increase in the inflammatory reactions having a very high quantity of cytokines and inflammatory biomarkers due to COVID-19 that were known to be managed by the beneficial use of corticosteroids.

Corticosteroids showed significant improvement in the patients who required number eight medical care, having shortness of breath as just in between 2-3 of getting infected, the internal secretion initiated and showed the prevention of acute biological conditions distress syndrome and even death. Corticosteroids like Deltasone or methylprednisolone (dose of 1 mg/kg equivalent per day), when taken along with some anti-viral agents, increased the internal secretion of plasma concentration and its half-life as well. The combination was taken for 3-4 weeks for effective results. This protocol resulted in the decline of proper anti-viral medicines, including(lopinavir and anti-viral agent (LPV/r) or darunavir and anti-viral agent (DRV/r)) and/or medicament, empirical broad-spectrum antibiotic treatment for fourteen days, and preventive medical care for 14–21 days. The formula of internal secretion treatment was used for severe pneumocystis carinii pneumonia besides forestall viscus pathology [16].

Interferons

Interferons are the cytokines that impart an essential role in inhibiting the multiplication of the host in the biological system of a human being. IFNs area unit free by plasmacytoid fiber cells throughout infection [17]. IFN has non-specific anti-viral effects, due to which it has been noticed effective in the treatment of MERS-CoV and SARS-CoV. INF has shown different results like lopinavir/ritonavir, ribavirin, remdesivir, corticosteroids, or IFNγ. IFN plays a crucial role in inflammation, immunomodulation, and signaling by activating the IFN-stimulated genes after binding to their receptors [18]. IFNs collectively sensitize cells of the human body to agent proteins to fend off agent fusion or egress. In vitro studies have shown that SARS-CoV-2 may be more sensitive to IFN than to the different COVID-19. Whereas INFs seemed to be economical for, in vitro and animal biological system models, they did not signify a valuable lead to patients with the disease.

HERBAL IMMUNOMODULATORS

Giloy (*Tinospora cordifolia*)

Giloy in Ayurvedic systems of medication has tremendous healthful blessings. It has been used for many years altogether for fever-reducing forms and purifies the blood, boost immunity, analgesic, medication, and anti-inflammatory blessings. It is used as a valuable remedy for the treatment of chronic cough, SOB, T.B., leprosy, syphilis, and venereal disease in Unani medication. Substances that are isolated from Tinosporacordifolia embrace polysaccharides, phenolics, diterpenoid, steroids, and sesquiterpenoids. Tinosporacordifolia holds radical scavenging property. Tinosporacordifolia reduces histamine-induced spasm in varied animal studies. One in each of the compounds, for, e.g., 1, 4-alpha-D-glucan derived from Tinosporacordifolia, has been known to start-off macrophages, NFκB translocation, and macromolecule production, and so activates the system [19]. Favorable effects of Tinosporacordifolia in HIV positive patients and Infectious sac malady in young chicks were exposed once it had been used with typical anti-viral treatment [20].

Ginger (*Zingiber officinale*)

It is sometimes used in old medication as a degree course and general tonic. The rootstock has been used for many years to treat upset, flatulence, high sign, arthritis, and the cold. It contains various bioactive ingredients like matter, zingiberine, shogaol, gingerdione, hexahydrocurcumin, paradol, and gingerenone A. keep with newer researches; ginger has very high levels of antioxidants that facilitate trim aerobic stress and suppress superoxide production. Extract of dried ginger has strong medicine and analgesic activities. It has been reportable having the most straightforward way higher impact against influenza (H1N1) and human biological process syncytial virus in human tract cell lines. Ginger also shows the bronchodilatory impact, prevents critical harm to the respiratory system thanks to inflammation, and improves allergic respiratory illness.

Black Pepper (*Piper nigrum*)

It is the same to be effective in fevers, SOB, asthma, different biological process diseases, bioactive components medicine, and antimicrobial properties, besides totally different blessings, considerably its marked bio-enhancing ability. It is a vital substance and radical scavenging properties.

Neem (*Azadirachta indica*)

It is used as antiseptic, blood equipment, antimicrobial, analgesic, antipyretic, (and medicine, and anti inflammatory) action significant plant. The bark and leaves unit is used for healthful functions. The various compounds are extracted from this herb include; Nimbin, Nimbin, nimbolide, limonoids, β-sitosterol, and quercitin. Scientific studies have proved its substance, medicine, immune-modulatory, medicine, antifungal, antipyretic, and antineoplastic activities. Along with the immunomodulatory operation, it has also been seen in in-vitro studies that it inhibits infectious agent replication and may be an influential agent for coxsackieviruses, herpes simplex virus type-1[21].

Turmeric (*Curcuma longa*)

Turmeric is a potent medicine used as an analgesic, antipyretic, blood equipment, and healing property. Scientists have reportable it to possess substance, immune-modulating, medicine, antimicrobial, and antitumor activities—the required ingredients of turmeric unit Curcumin, dihydro curcumin, and hexahydrocurcumin [22]. Cineol, α-phellandrene, borneol, zingiberine, and all different sesquiterpenes are some of the volatile compounds found in turmeric [23]. Curcumin has been determined to work in acute biological process distress syndrome, COPD, acute internal organ injury, and pneumonic pathology. Turmeric subdues the TNF-α and inhibits NF-κB; in this way, it acts as a potent medicine. Monocot genus extract acts against varied unhealthful organisms at the side of strep, cocci, *Klebsiella pneumonia*, *Helicobacter pylori*, *Bacillus subtilis*, eubacteria *Asiatic cholera*, etc.

Garlic (*Allium sativum*)

Garlic has many active ingredients at the side of alliin, allicin, ajoene, vinyldithin, S-allyl organic compound, and diallyl sulfides. A more than studies discovered garlic to possess substance, medicine, immune-modulating, antibiotic, organic process, antifungal, anti-viral, antihelminthic, antithrombic, hypotensive, hypoglycemic, and hypo-cholesterolemic properties. Extract of garlic shows potent anti-viral action against respiratory illness, herpes simplex, and coxsackieviruses. Extract of garlic reduces the migration of polymorphonuclear cells through epithelium cell layers. It suppresses the assembly of gas and prostaglandin-E2, subdues the inducible variety of gas synthase and cyclooxygenase expression, and reduces the assembly of various inflammatory cytokines TNF-α, cytokine half-dozen, and medicine.

Cinnamon (*Cinnamomum zeylanicum*)

It has been used for many years in treating biological process ailments like cough and respiratory illness besides having antiseptic, cardiotonic, aphrodisiac, and phlegmagogue actions. To boot, researchers have found this herb effective in genetic disorders, Alzheimer's malady, anemia, heart diseases, dyslipidemia, upset, and stomachal cancer to its medicine, substance, and antimicrobial properties. The active ingredients in the cinnamon unit are cinnamic acid, cinnamaldehyde, cinnamate, and diverse essential oils like eugenol, trans-cinnamaldehyde, cinnamyl acetate, caryophyllene compound, L-borneol, E-nerolidol, b-caryophyllene, α-thujene, α-cubebene, α-terpinol, and terpinolene. The extract nanoparticles from the bark were proved to possess degree anti-viral impact, inhibiting the activity of H7N3 respiratory illness an outbreak in Vero cells.

Amla (*Emblica officinalis*)

Amla is bitter and is the richest source of inhibitor. The fruit of amla is improbably used for healthful functions. These surprise fruit choices an effective alternative to activities and may treat several ailments [24]. It is used to treat colds, fever, dyspepsia, hair growth, liver disorders, etc. Amla contains inhibitor, iron, calcium, and diverse bioactive various compounds like acid, ellagic acid, nonsesquiterpenoids, geranium, and prodelphinidins. Various preclinical studies have discovered amla as a potent substance and have anti-inflammatory, immune attention, radical scavenger, antipyretic, medication, hematinic, hepatoprotective, neuroprotective, and antitumor properties in it. Due to its extreme immune empowering property, it is known to have properties that are against infections. It is effective against cold, bronchitis, influenza conditions and shows increased refinement in AIDS and cancer patients. It is derived from black pepper embrace piperine, piperic acid, piperamide, piperlonguminine, piperolein-B, pellitorine, piperidine, eugenol, and kusonokinin, in addition to some volatile oils—multiple in-vitro and in-vivo studies units administered to prove substance.

NIH Guidelines for the Treatment of COVID-19 by Immunomodulators

The COVID-19 Treatments Guidelines Panel prepared various guidelines to follow for everyone in the medical management of COVID-19 external icons published by the National Institutes of Health. The guidelines include various information about medicinal therapeutics, the drugs, and various therapeutic interference that FDA approves for use.

Various drugs and medicaments were suggested for use in the treatment or prevention of the COVID-19 virus. Those drugs and their clinical trials are still being studied to be used later if approved.

The COVID-19 Treatment Guidelines Panel is regularly working on the latest reviews and clinical data so that updated treatment can be given to the patients suffering from COVID-19. The panel provides the information for the management of patients according to their severity of disease because some patients show mild symptoms whereas some patients show severe symptoms. These guidelines also provide clinical data of the drugs and medicaments going under investigation in Anti-viral therapy, Immune-based therapy, and Adjunctive therapy sections.

Recommendations

The panel does not endorse any particular drug, even if it is anti-viral or immunomodulatory therapy, for the treatment of COVID 19 patients, no matter if they are not hospitalized or hospitalized with mild symptoms without supplemental oxygen. If the patient has an oxygen level ≥of 94% on room air at sea level, the patient is contemplating having moderate disease and symptoms and has clinical and radiographic evidence of lower respiratory tract infection. The panel has no sufficient data for the utilization of the drug Remdesivir in the therapy of COVID-19. The panel has also endorsed not to use corticosteroids like Dexamethasone for COVID 19 treatment until the patient has any other reason (disease) for its use.

Additional Considerations

It is acknowledged by the panel that there were situations in which clinicians judged that Remdesivir is a suitable therapy for a patient who is hospitalized with moderate disease (e.g., a person who is at exceptionally high risk for clinical deterioration). If the patient is at a high risk of having clinical collapse, then the panel may recommend the clinicians and doctors for the use of Remdesivir, but only if the person is hospitalized with moderate disease. The rationale for Not Endorsing Routine Use of Remdesivir in the Group of Patients. During the Adaptive COVID 19 Treatment Trial (ACTT-1), a multinational, arbitrary trial was held between Remdesivir and placebo in the patients suffering from hospitalized with mild to even moderate symptoms. However, there was no benefit shown for Remdesivir (defined as SpO_2>94% on room air or a respiratory rate <24 breaths/min without supplemental oxygen) [25].

Ministry of AYUSH Recommendation

Some self-help directions for preventing various health measures and gearing-up immunity with particular reference to respiratory health are given in this section.

1. Wide-ranging events for enhancing immunity:
    - Use warm water
    - Ministry of AYUSH advises everyone to do meditation and yoga.
    - Make a regular habit of taking spice like *Haldi* (Turmeric), *Jeera* (Cumin), *Dhania* (Coriander), and *Lehsuna* (Garlic) are suggested in cooking.
2. Immunity Promoting by Ayurveda:
    - Take *Chyavanprasha* in the morning; sugar-free *Chyavanprasha* gave to diabetes people.
    - Once or twice a day, drink herbal tea/ decoction (*Kadha*) made from *Tulsi*, *Dalchini, Kalimirch*, *Shunthi*, and *Munnaka*. Add Jaggery and fresh Lemon juice for your taste.
    - Golden Milk prepares with *Haldi* (Turmeric) powder in hot milk.
3. Simple *Ayurvedic* Procedures:
    - Nasal Application- Bear on sesame oil/ coconut oil or *Ghee* in both the nostrils (*PratimarshNasya*) in the morning and evening.
    - *Kaval* (Oil Pulling) Therapy- Take one tablespoon of sesame or coconut oil in the mouth. Do not drink; swish in the mouth for two to 3 minutes and spit it off, followed by a warm water rinse once or twice a day.
4. Precaution during symptoms like dry cough/ sore throat:
    - Fresh *Pudina* (Mint) leaves or *Ajwain* (Caraway seeds) steam inhalation used.
    - During cough or throat irritation, make a habit of using *Lavang*powder assorted with natural sugar/ honey can be taken 2-3 times a day.

- Though, if these symptoms persist even taken above measure, then it is best to consult doctors.

5. Precautionary measures: When an infected person sneezes or coughs and their respiratory droplets are ejected into the air, coronavirus is spread. These few drops can persist in the nasal area and mouth of others within 6 feet, causing the virus to spread. To decrease the contamination, basic safety protocols should be following as we know coronavirus is highly transmittable:
   - Regularly wash the hands.
   - Sanitize hands and frequently touched surfaces with sanitizers.
   - Avoid touching the eyes, nose, and mouth with unwashed hands.
   - During sneezing, make use of tissue paper or use your elbow.
   - Stay safe and stay home.
   - Stay alone if a member of your family is sick.
   - Make a habit of using a mask when you are sick or in a crowded area.
   - Maintain social distance.
   - Avoid unnecessary traveling.

Conclusion

This structured review showed that the therapies based on the immunomodulation are encouraging and also gave a valuable therapeutic policy to the scientific community and clinicians so that they can fight back against this outbreak pandemic in no time because other approaches like vaccines and medicines may come into the use only in the future. If the patients have a difficult or critical situation due to COVID-19, then immunomodulator therapy should be used immediately within the time.

REFERENCES

[1] World Health Organization. Clinical management of severe acute respiratory infection (SARI) when COVID-19 disease is suspected. *Interim guidance*. 13 March 2020.

[2] Akshat Agrawal, Rajesh Arora, Ranjna Arora, Prateek Agrawal. (2021). Applications of Artificial Intelligence and Internet of Things for Detection and Future Directions to Fight against COVID-19. In edited book on *Emerging Technologies for Battling Covid-19*, pp. 107-119, Springer.

[3] V Madaan, A Roy, C Gupta, P Agrawal, A Sharma, C Bologa, R Prodan. (2021). XCOVNet: Chest X-ray Image Classification for COVID-19 Early Detection Using Convolutional Neural Networks. *New Generation Computing*, pp. 1-15, 2021. doi: 10.1007/ s00354-021-00121-7.

[4] Prateek Agrawal, Vishu Madaan, Aditya Roy, Rajani Kumari & Harshal Deore. (2021). FOCOMO: Forecasting and monitoring the worldwide spread of COVID-19 using machine learning methods, *Journal of Interdisciplinary Mathematics*, pp. 1-25. doi: 10.1080/09720502.2021.1885812.

[5] Webster NR, Galley HF. Immunomodulation in the critically ill. *Br J Anaesth*. 2009;103(1):70–81. https://doi.org/10.1093/bja/aep 128.

[6] Busse, KH., E. Formentini, RM. Alfaro, JA. Kovacs, SR. PenzakInfluence of antiretroviral drugs on the pharmacokinetics of prednisolone in HIV-infected individuals, *J Acquir Immune DeficSyndr*, 48 (2008), pp. 561-566.

[7] Bozzette, SA., FR. Sattler, J. Chiu, AW. Wu, D. Gluckstein, C. Kemper, et al. A controlled trial of early adjunctive treatment with corticosteroids for *Pneumocystis carinii* pneumonia in the acquired immunodeficiency syndrome, *N Engl J Med*, 323 (1990), pp. 1451-1457.

[8] Sallard E, Lescure FX, Yazdanpanah Y, Mentre F, Peiffer-Smadja N. Type 1 interferons as a potential treatment against COVID-19. *Antiviral Res*. 2020;178:104791.

[9] Merad M, Martin JC. Pathological inflammation in patients with COVID-19: a key role for monocytes and macrophages [published

correction appears in *Nat Rev Immunol*. 2020;20(7):448]. *Nat Rev Immunol*. 2020;20(6):355–62.
[10] Richardson P, Griffin I, Tucker C, et al. Baricitinib as potential treatment for 2019-nCoV acute respiratory disease. *Lancet*. 2020;395(10223):e30–e3131.
[11] Casadevall A, Pirofski L. The convalescent sera option for containing COVID-19. *J Clin Investig*. 2020;130:1545–8.
[12] Umapathi T, Kor AC, Venketasubramanian N, et al. Large artery ischaemic stroke in severe acute respiratory syndrome (SARS). *J Neurol*. 2004;251:1227–311.
[13] Shang L, Zhao J, Hu Y, et al. On the use of corticosteroids for 2019-nCoV pneumonia. *Lancet*. 2020;395:683–4.
[14] Khosa RL, Prasad S. Pharmacognostical studies on Guduchi (*Tinospora cordifolia* Miers) *J Res Ind Med*. 1971;6:261–9.
[15] Prince PS, Kamalakkannan N, Menon VP. Restoration of antioxidants by ethanolic *Tinospora cordifolia* in alloxan-induced diabetic Wistar rats. *Acta Pol Pharm*. 2004; 61:283–7.
[16] Denyer CV, Jackson P, Loakes DM, Ellis MR, Young DA. Isolation of antirhinoviral sesquiterpenes from ginger (*Zingiber officinale*). *J Nat Prod*. 1994; 57(5):658-662. Weekly Epidemiological Update Data as received by WHO from national authorities, as of 10 am CEST 6 September 2020.
[17] Tiwari V, Darmani NA, Yue BY, Shukla D. In vitro anti-viral activity of neem (*Azadirachta indica* L.) bark extract against herpes simplex virus type-1 infection. *Phytother Res*. 2013; 24(8):1132-1140.
[18] Hewlings SJ, Kalman DS. Curcumin: A review of its effects on human health. *Foods*. 2017; 6(10): 92.
[19] Nayampalli S, Ainapure SS, Nadkarni PM. Study of antiallergic acid Bronchodilator effects of *Tinospora cordifolia*. *Indian J Pharmacol*. 1982;14:64–6.
[20] Nayampalli SS, Desai NK, Ainapure SS. Anti-allergic properties of *Tinospora cordifolia* in animal models. *Indian J Pharmacol*. 1986; 18:250–2.
[21] Shang A, Cao SY, Xu XY, et al. Bioactive compounds and biological functions of garlic (*Allium sativum* L.). *Foods*. 2019; 8(7):246. doi:10.3390/foods8070246.

[22] Niamsa N, Sittiwet C. Antimicrobial activity of *Curcuma longa* aqueous extract. *Journal of Pharmacology and Toxicology*. 2009; 4(4):173–177.
[23] Rao PV, Gan SH. Cinnamon: a multifaceted medicinal plant. *Evid Based Complement Alternat Med*. 2014; 2014:642942. dio: 10.1155/2014/642942.
[24] Baliga MS, Dsouza JJ. Amla (*Emblica officinalis* Gaertn), a wonder berry in the treatment and prevention of cancer. *Eur J Cancer Prev.* 2011; 20(3):225-239.
[25] Beigel JH, Tomashek K, Dodd L, et al. Remdesivir for the treatment of COVID-19—final report. *N Engl J Med*. 2020; Published online ahead of print.

In: Impacts and Implications of COVID-19 ISBN: 978-1-53619-670-2
Editors: Anand Sharma et al.

Chapter 3

Development of Social Distancing Detection Tool for COVID-19

Vibha Ojha[1,*], Divya Sharma[2] and Anand Sharma[3]
[1]Govt. Engineering College, Ajmer, India
[2]Govt. Engineering College, Bikaner, India
[3]School of Engineering and Technology, MUST, Lakshmangarh, India

Abstract

COVID-19, a disease that has brought the world down these days. A destructive infection is spreading among individuals at a rapid rate. One of the ways to stop its spread is by keeping a social distance. Social distancing, which we also say actual distancing, obviously implies keeping a proper distance between two individuals who are not from a similar family. The ideal approach to rehearse social distancing is to remain at 6 feet from others.

Social distancing is a significant way to decrease the spread of irresistible illnesses. This is a typical practice that has been used over ages to limit the spread of infection by restricting its spreading rate amid communities. People from various families are approached to keep their communications with one another less,

---

* Corresponding Author's E-mail: vibha.ojha@gmail.com.

which will help diminish the odds of the illness being spread among individuals and, consequently, will guarantee just that social distancing convention out in the open spots. The working environment is kept up or not; this section is centered around building up a social distancing detection tool that can screen if individuals are staying away from one another by investigating ongoing video transfers from the camera utilizing OpenCV.

Keywords: COVID-19, coronavirus, WHO, social distancing, OpenCV

Introduction

The present outburst of the coronavirus or COVID-19 was articulated as an overall wellbeing emergency by the WHO. More than one million people have been affected by this infection, with more than 50000 people have died to date.

A declared 200 countries have reported examples of COVID-19 in which the United States has the most significant number of cases and Italy has the most fatalities due to this infection [1, 2].

The earnestness of the disease goes from asymptomatic to lethal stages by and prominent impacting people with a frail safe framework and the more established people. COVID-19 shifts from SARS-COV where patients in the prodromal period can deliver a colossal proportion of contamination replications adding to the spread of the diseases.

In SARS-COV patients, transmission happened just when serious ailment was noticed, making it simpler to be identified as not usual for COVID-19 [3]. The transmission is overwhelmingly recognized as through droplets and airborne transmission. Few examinations are being directed over COVID-19 in air tests, and WHO has not distinguished the illness as an airborne sickness to date [4].

A dominant part of the patients is tried just if the indications are appeared by them, subsequently making it less dependable to recognize the number of "hidden deaths" brought about by Coronavirus [5]. The requirement for testing has been worried by the WHO consistently with the absence of test packs and personal protective equipment (PPE) in a few nations; there is a high possibility that a great deal of patients experiencing COVID-19 goes undetected [6, 7].

SOCIAL DISTANCING

This section shows the significance of social distancing during the COVID-19 outburst. Social distancing, lockdown, and sanitization have been used and heard by almost everyone in a few nations. At first, the lockdown or shutting down everything except necessities was imposed in Wuhan, China, to decrease the spread of the sickness to different parts of the country and continuously different nations, for example, Germany, Italy, Sri Lanka, Israel, Belgium, India, UK, and France began to follow a similar interaction.

Social distancing is a method to limit the physical contact of people and reduce the spread of sickness among individuals. This is a typical practice used overages, for example, the understudy and educator co-operations where almost all understudies try not to be nearest to the instructor and lean toward remaining in the last columns [8]. During the influenza pandemic in 1918, a detailed 50 to 100 million people died worldwide; albeit social distancing was not executed, a more significant part of the populace took "receptive social distancing measures" that made it conceivable to get away from the illness outbreak [9]. This practice, followed by a few million people, prompted the pandemic restricting the harm after world war one out of a few European nations. Similarly, during 1957-58, the H2N2 infection (Asia Flu) infected many people, and Asians were restricted to traverse lines and stays inside during the pandemic [10]. As of late ten years prior, the outbreak of H1N1, otherwise called pig influenza, influenced almost 60 million people. The spread of the sickness was controlled utilizing general estimates, for example, social distancing to maintain a strategic distance from the human-to-human transmission of the illness [11].

Social-distance is a social-science idea. It alludes to the sentiments of 'lack of approachability&unapproachably capacity', particularly amidst individuals from various social layers [12]. It is rehearsed, taking all things together social orders in fluctuating degrees. The idea was promoted about a century ago by Emory S Bogardus in the USA. He saw that 'social distances exist among various gatherings of individuals just as among people's and its 'boss importance' is to look after status [13]. However, social distancing, as a general wellbeing measure during pandemics, has been animated by works during the Middle Ages. Lipton and Steinhauer compose that social distancing turned out to be essential for the government strategy of the USA about ten years prior [14]. It was utilized limitedly during the H1N1 flu outbreak in 2009.

In the present COVID-19 pandemic, the social distancing has been executed across the USA interestingly. Though social distancing has turned into USA government strategy lately, it has been rehearsed for quite a while at this point. It has been a new focal point of examination too. In the USA, during the 1918 flu pandemic, urban communities seeing the early presentation of social-distancing and different mediations had decreased top passing rates and less steep scourge bends [15]. Demonstrating examines been strong of social-distancing in a thorough audit of displaying and epidemiological investigations on social-distancing in non-healthcare work environments. The proof is arising on social-distancing in the present COVID-19 pandemic, and it has been remarked that the logical premise and moral contemplation of such mediation should be considered [16].

The impacts of social distancing as a general wellbeing measure in controlling pestilences are becoming known. Its impacts on human social orders are not too seen, however. Nor has it been seen what cultural changes set off by social distancing can mean for general wellbeing. Social distancing is probably going to be unpleasant, particularly for more established grown-ups. Human interaction dependent on computerized digital innovation is probably going to increment.

Social Distancing at Home

- As referenced, practice great hand and sniffle/hack cleanliness;
- Increase ventilation in the home by opening windows or changing cooling;
- Regularly sanitize high touch surfaces, for example, tables, kitchen seats, and door handles;
- Avoid kissing and handshaking;
- Visit shops sparingly and purchase more products and enterprises on the web;
- Keep the way to the debilitated individual's room shut and, if conceivable, a window open;

- Care for the sick individual in a solitary room if conceivable;
- Consider whether trips and travel, both individual and family, are reasonable and vital;
- Both the debilitated individual and individuals focusing on them should wear a surgical mask when they are in a similar room;
- Protect other weak relatives, for example, individuals more than 65 years or individuals with an ongoing ailment, including, if practicable, discovering elective convenience.

Social-Distancing in the Workplace

- Avoid in-person gatherings. Utilize email facility, online conferencing, or the telephone whenever the situation allows, in any event, when individuals are in a similar building. Unavoidable in-person gatherings ought to be short in timings, in large meeting rooms where individuals can sit at least 6 feet from one another; try not to shake hands;
- Do not gather in workrooms, copier rooms, storerooms, or different regions where individuals socialize;
- Eliminate superfluous travel& drop or postpone non-essential meetings, social occasions, training meetings, and workshops;
- Bring lunch and eat at your work area or away from others;
- Avoid public transportation and used-car, cycle or walk or go early or late to stay away from busy times at public places;
- Limit sporting or other recreation classes, activities, meetings, and so on, where close contact with others is likely.

Social Distancing in Schools

- If the child is debilitated, do not send them to class (or childcare);
- Defer exercises that lead to blending among classes and years;
- Sanities hands when entering school and at standard stretches;
- Avoid lining and consider dropping school congregations;
- Conduct exercises outside where conceivable;

- Clean and sterilize high touch surfaces consistently;
- Promote a regular hand-washing plan;
- Consider opening windows and changing molding for more ventilation;
- Promote the strictest cleanliness among food readiness staff and their nearby contacts.

Social Distancing in Public

- Use tap and pay instead of taking care of cash;
- Sanitize hands at every possible opportunity, including entering and leaving buildings;
- Public vehicle laborers and cabbies should open vehicle windows conceivable and routinely perfect and purify high touch surfaces;
- Try and travel on casual occasions and attempt to dodge swarms.

Importance of Social-Distancing Practices

Social-distancing assimilates approaches to stop or decrease the spread of infections. It promotes less contact among people. Social distancing is essential because COVID-19 tends to spread from individual to individual through:

- direct close contact with an individual while they are irresistible or in the 24 hours before their indications showed up,
- touching articles or surfaces (for example, tables, chairs, or door handles or) polluted from a hack or sniffle from an individual with an affirmed contamination, and afterward contacting your mouth or face,
- close contact with an individual with an affirmed contamination who hacks or sniffles.

Thus, the probability of spreading the infection will decrease if the people are physically distanced from one another.

In the advanced world, connections are made on a standard premise utilizing innovation accessible yet more extensive part exercises completed consistently depends on social communication. Social communication and contact are vital as an efficient point of view for the country as laborers need to work consistently to permit income in their separate organizations; it is additionally a fundamental piece of dealers and customers to produce income [17].

A social distancing practice permits people to keep up good ways from one another for a while to guarantee the spread of the sickness is limited. This would lessen the essential propagation pace of the infection, which would limit the illness spread. Prem et al. [18] investigated that if social-distancing rehearses are done appropriately, a gauge of 92% of cases is brought down toward the finish of 2020.

A person infected with COVID-19 can spread the infection to 2-3 people who will further spread it until they are physically distanced from one other. There are two common practices that are followed using social distancing; one of them is social distancing and maintaining a distance of nearly 1meter from one another, and the other is staying at home. This practice has been successful in the past and the present as well, where Wuhan was able to flatten the disease spread by following these practices. This method does not need any cost and entirely dependent on the behavior of individuals, where most of them do not abide by the rules put out in the country [19].

If social-distancing methods have been ignored, then the effect could last on for the upcoming generations as the COVID-19 virus will develop different strains where to date, eight different strains of the virus have been discovered by scientists.

On the off chance that social distancing strategies are overlooked, the impact could keep going on for the forthcoming ages as the COVID-19 infection will want to create various strains. As of date, eight distinct strains of the infection have been found by researchers [20].

IMPACT OF SOCIAL DISTANCING

On Children

To decrease the spread of diseases, many schools are shut the nation over, influencing students, their gatekeepers, and guardians. It has interfered with the youngsters' schooling and has influenced families past it. As per the Centers for Disease Control and Prevention (CDC), understudies that rely upon the school administrations for supper projects and social, physical, and psychological wellbeing administrations will be influenced in light of the delayed conclusion of schools. Emotional wellness issues may likewise increment among youngsters because of diminished freedoms to draw in with peers. Effectively actual broken conduct found in youths may be exasperated in the pandemic, and with the conclusion of schools, understudies will not have a comparative way to deal with the psychological wellness organizations. Studies show that teenagers from the age of 12 to 17 have been analyzed with nervousness or discouragement. Implosion is one of the significant danger factors among teenagers [21].

On Substance Users

Individuals with substance use disorders (SUD) have a high chance of getting contaminated due to various components inferable from their mental, clinical and crazy conditions. Moreover, social and monetary changes achieved by the pandemic, close by the challenges as for treatment approach and adherence-which will certainly increment during this time, thus forward additional upsetting their condition. To measure the impact of COVID on substance clients and to suggest specific frameworks, it is crucial to consider the qualities of these developments, for instance, a) people with mellow SUD versus moderate to severe SUD; b) those presently into restraint versus dynamic substance use; c) those with co-sullen mental issues (counting usage of different substances). Individuals with moderate to severe SUD are currently huge danger gathering and could struggle extreme impacts since they have been identified with all of these sicknesses. Moreover, previous a few investigations have declared that tobacco and alcohol ingestion can incite flu. Substance clients who regularly abuse the substances in a blend of various medications can cause added hazards. While substance use can enlarge the dangers identified with COVID pollution, the social and mental chance of the pandemic can raise substance use in a dangerous cycle. Actual distance, quarantine, or confinement are essential systems to end sickness transmission — in any case, the procedures, and the pandemic, has been connected with hostile antagonism, for instance, anxiety, crabbiness, wretchedness, shock, uneasiness, or weariness.

Withdrawal signs motivated during seclusion could in like manner jeopardize these security procedures, as individuals could venture out searching for drugs. Moreover, clinical assistance for signs will be limited since the vast clinical undertakings are equipped towards the COVID-19 pandemic. Besides, these people can be possible transmitters for contamination. Express procedures for anticipation and treatment should be discussed. Healthcare laborers overseeing SUD ought to think about the troubles they should look at during and after the COVID-19 outbreak [22].

On the Geriatric Population

Older adults are more plausible to build up some genuine mental problems than people of different ages because they get contaminated with the COVID. Due to their great danger to the contamination, it is especially critical for them to keep up physical distancing amid the wide range of various defensive measures. These defensive measures can control them from having associations with their companions, guardians, and family, which could incite extended sensation of anxiety and dejection. Moreover, the general sensation of weakness and danger gave a pandemic. More seasoned people have a high possibility of sadness, which is now misidentified and untreated in this general population.

The recurrence of bitterness and stress increases among people who need home medical services or individuals who require emergency clinic therapies. Implosion is a related enthusiastic danger among the geriatric populace [23].

On Overall Population

Social distancing will no doubt expand anxiety, fear, melancholy, and depression. People are social animals, liberated from ethnicity, and keeping up distance for quite a while may create critical mental pressure. The monetary weight during the pandemic, with huge unemployment, increment in penury, awkwardness, may accentuate such emotions. Impacts are extraordinary in evolved nations for — the people in healthcare offices, the transients, and people with crazy issues. A US-based examination investigated more than 10 million Google look and assessed the progressions in mental health inquiries after the lockdown orders [24].

Implications for Public Health

The immediate and most perceived impact of social distancing on general wellbeing is its capacity to restrain the spread of a scourge. Disease transmission experts' opinion in this regard is that the spread of COVID-19 cannot be halted. Nonetheless, it very well may be eased back down impressively by receiving social-distancing measures. By restricting physical contact, the rate of transmission can be diminished considerably, increasing the time to spread it. With COVID-19 expected to keep going for quite a long time, and immunizations and medications are now inaccessible, social distancing should be noticed for an extended period. The far-reaching practice of telemedicine is relied upon to decrease topographical imbalances in admittance to healthcare. The various changes achieved by enormous scope adherence to social distancing rules have a few different ramifications for general wellbeing in India. Specifically, such changes will affect the socio-social determinants of human conduct. The changed thought of personal space (and protection) can ameliorate the prevalent practices at healthcare facilities. Security maintenance in such settings can be undermined in the country. This is particularly obvious on account of socio-monetarily impeded individuals. An altered thought of personal space will raise the assumptions for patients from their healthcare suppliers. The last mentioned, then again, will be more aware of ensuring the protection of the patients. Similarly, keeping up the distance between people while undertaking general wellbeing research (e.g., surveys on wellbeing) might be standard.

What will be the impact of the changing idea of regular great on general wellbeing in India? Public wellbeing is established in the thought of typical great. It is pitched to achieve positive changes at the populace level. General wellbeing gains are cultural and not individuated accounts of care and recuperation. Rehearsing social distancing is as much a measure to shield himself/herself from the infection for what it is worth about shielding others from oneself. It is an action that advances the benefit of everyone. It is an uncommon event when conduct alteration in the populace is so enthusiastic in nations across the globe.

Terms, for example, "do your part, stay separated," and 'social distancing are getting instilled in the well-known creative mind. Deviations, in any case, are the push to the group to rehearse social distancing and its adherence by individuals that will help the preventive parts of public health. The tweaking of sexual orientation jobs in the family unit would be advantageous for ladies' physical and psychological wellbeing. Be that as it may, this would be conceivable just if ladies and young ladies lead a daily existence liberated from viciousness. The changed sexual orientation jobs combined with a viciousness-free life would help ladies' wellbeing looking for conduct. Women experience job strain and have little recreation because of the different weights of childcare and family obligations and paid work. This influences their consideration of looking for conduct. The tweaking of sexual orientation parts in the family will probably offer them an opportunity to look for care.

Additionally, if telecommuting (or flexible working hours) turns into the new standard for some callings resulting from COVID-19, men would be sharing family unit duties. Indeed, even male association in ladies' wellbeing might be relied upon to increment because of more noteworthy sensitization achieved by long periods of sharing duties. It will probably bring about more evident appreciation for the neglected/came up short on family tasks ordinarily done by ladies and improve the poise agreed to such work.

PROPOSED SOCIAL DISTANCE DETECTION TOOL

Social distance detection between people on foot is accomplished in this work from monocular pictures without taking additional data is conceivable. One way which we can say is not exact is by asking the client for explicit information sources that ought to be prompting a distance assessment or figuring between the two. If the client could check any two of the given focuses on the showed outline that ought to be 6 feet separated, at that point utilizing extrapolation, one could without much of a stretch discover the distance that should be kept up between various focuses on the This would have been conceivable in the equipment project if we could put the camera at some equidistant to all the stamped focuses on the given plane where the nearer individuals are to the camera, the greater they would have shown upon it. We can likewise say that the nearer the two focuses are on the casing to the put camera, the more fair the actual distance would be in the middle of them, which will give us a bad outcome and, thus, the framework will be wasted.

To manage this issue, we build up this tool, which will recognize social distancing in a video. We will be giving four focuses as a contribution as the client to stamp those two lines that would be seen equal from above. The region that we would be set apart by these four focuses will be considered a region of interest (ROI). This is a polygon formed. This ROI will be distorted into a square shape that will be utilized to turn into the superior view. This birds-eye view is exceptionally successful as it has the property of focuses in which a similar number of pixels is separated from one another or, say, are being equidistant any place they are. All we require now is a multiplier that will be utilized to map the distance between two focuses in every pixel in the distance, all things considered, units like, for instance, in feet or meters.

The idea is utilized in this research is deep learning, which is essentially used to identify, detect and confine individuals that will be then planned in bird's eye view projection screen. When we get the ideal coordinates of individuals through the assistance of bird's eye view, at that point, the social distancing boundaries that we need will turn out to be straightforward.

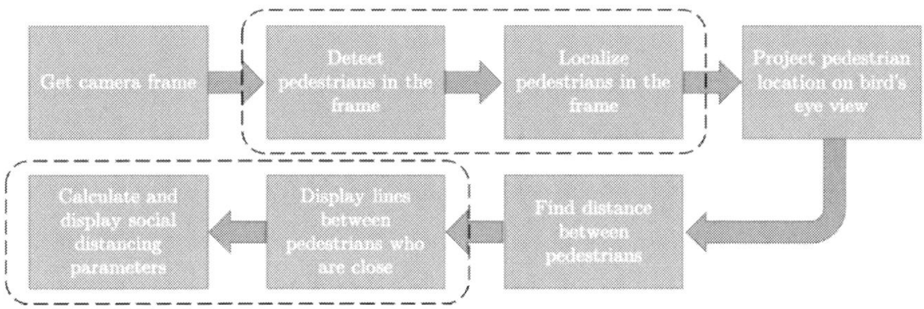

Figure 1. Workflow of proposed social distance detection tool.

This work is done in python utilizing OpenCV. OpenCV is one of the libraries which is fundamentally utilized for live undertaking or vision-related ventures.

OpenCV, as the name as of now states, represents Computer Vision. Its emphasis is on applications like picture handling, catching recordings, and investigation that incorporates some astounding highlights like face location and item recognition. Computer vision, or say OpenCVis fundamentally the development of explicit, is likewise a significant portrayal of actual items available in the picture. Essentially, the yield that we get from PC vision is the portrayal of an understanding of designs in a 3D manner. Thus, the job of this library is to identify the people on edge in the video. The platform on which we were doing our work is Anaconda Navigator. Boa constrictor Navigator is one of the most utilized work area applications. Primarily, it is a graphical UI (GUI). It causes us to utilize different applications and is utilized to oversee conda package, environment effectively Jupyter Notebook is one of the uses of a boa constrictor guide. It is usually an open-source web application.

Python language has been utilized in this work. Python is one of the late most utilized programming languages. It is, in like manner, an undeniable level programming language and one of a broadly functional programming language too.

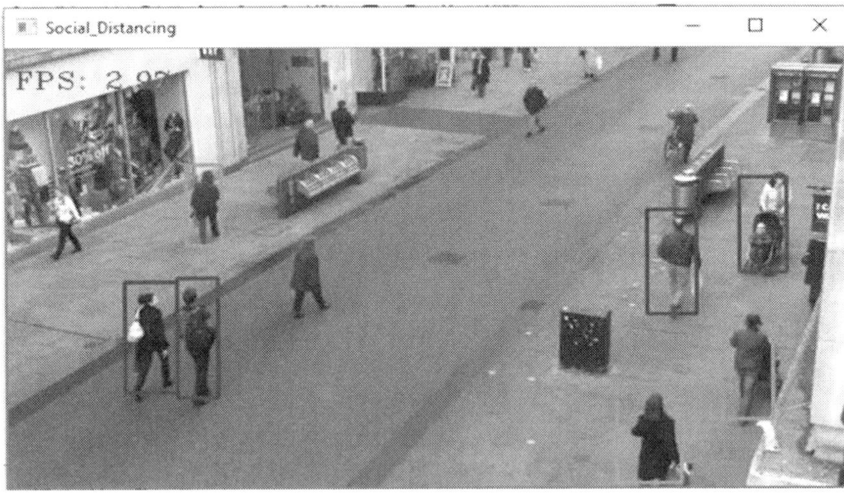

Figure 2. The output of social distance detection tool (Red block: High risk, Green block: Low or not at risk).

We tried our framework on an anaconda navigator. Our code was effectively ready to run here. Anaconda navigator guide is extraordinary compared to other work area applications for accomplishing machine learning work as it furnishes us with numerous libraries which we can straightforwardly import from the anaconda repository and use proficiently. We had the option to handily import libraries required for our work. Those were Scikitlearn, NumPy, Pandas, Matplotlib, and Seaborn. We utilized Jupyter Notebook for creating a social distance detection tool.

CONCLUSION

With the worldwide instances of raising the cases of COVID-19, the requirement for testing packs and PPE for healthcare laborers ought to become the most critical need for each nation to restrict and detect the sickness early. Additionally, mental and social help should be given during this time of isolation through online gateways to people experiencing despondency and loneliness and communication lines to forestall emotional wellbeing problems. Finally, we must remain aware of COVID-19 and report the indications and signs present, if any, to health authorities, instead of shroud it. Keeping up social distancing for a while will reduce the spread of illness.

Significant occasions achieve changes in the public arena. Social-distancing measures are required to be set up for a supported timeframe to restrict the spread of COVID-19. Keeping up social distancing is presumably to become propensity framing, with its belongings working out positively past restricting the spread of the infection. The use and encouragement of social distancing at different spots (e.g., workplaces, instructive foundations) and in different ways will probably make it standard in the Indian culture. People are social creatures. During these challenging and difficult times, innovation has made it workable for us to remain associated and get healthcare in innovative courses regardless of rehearsing social distancing. This makes the experience an alternate one than what would have been the situation in before times.

After using this tool, we were effectively ready to identify who was keeping up social distancing and who was not. In the video, the person who was at a safe distance appeared with the green shading box's assistance. However, the closed person appeared with the assistance of a red shading box. Red shading box individuals are more inclined to get contaminated by the sickness, while the one encompassed by green tone is less likely to get tainted.

REFERENCES

[1] https://www.google.com/covid19-map/

[2] Agrawal, Prateek, Madaan, Vishu, Roy, Aditya, Kumari, Rajani, Deore, Harshal (2021). FOCOMO: Forecasting and monitoring the worldwide spread of COVID-19 using machine learning methods, *Journal of Interdisciplinary Mathematics*, pp. 1-25. DOI: 10.1080/09720502.2021.1885812

[3] Lipsitch, M., Swerdlow, D.L. and Finelli, L., 2020. Defining the epidemiology of Covid-19—studies needed. *New England Journal of Medicine*.

[4] https://www.who.int/newsroom/commentaries/detail/modes-oftransmission-of-virus-causing-covid-19-implications-for-ipc-precautionrecommendations.

[5] Agrawal, Akshat, Arora, Rajesh, Arora, Ranjna, Agrawal, Prateek(2021). Applications of Artificial Intelligence and Internet of Things for Detection and Future Directions to Fight Against COVID-19. In an edited book on *Emerging Technologies for Battling Covid-19*, pp. 107-119, Springer.

[6] Madaan, V., Roy, A., Gupta, C., Agrawal, P., Sharma, A., Bologa, C., Prodan, R. (2021). XCOVNet: Chest X-ray Image Classification for COVID-19 Early Detection Using Convolutional Neural Networks. *New Generation Computing*, pp. 1-15, 2021. DOI: 10.1007/ s00354-021-00121-7.

[7] Vetter, P., Eckerle, I. and Kaiser, L., 2020. *Covid-19: A puzzle with many missing pieces*.

[8] Schwebel, A.I. and Cherlin, D.L., 1972. Physical and social distancing in teacher-pupil relationships. *Journal of Educational Psychology*, 63(6), p.543.

[9] Yu, D., Lin, Q., Chiu, A.P. and He, D., 2017. Effects of reactive social distancing on the 1918 influenza pandemic. *PloS one*, 12(7).

[10] Jackson, C., 2009. History lessons: the Asian Flu pandemic. *Br J Gen Pract*, 59(565), pp.622-623.

[11] Sebastian, M.R., Lodha, R. and Kabra, S.K., 2009. Swine origin influenza (swine flu). *The Indian Journal of Pediatrics*, 76(8), p.833.

[12] Jary, D., &Jary, J., 1991.*Collins dictionary of sociology*. Harper Collins Publishers.

[13] Bogardus, E. S., 1926. Social distance in the city. *Proceedings and Publications of the American Sociological Society, 20,* 40–46. https://brocku.ca/MeadProject/Bogardus/Bogardus_1926.html

[14] Lipton, E., &Steinhauer, J., 2020. The untold story of the birth of social distancing. *The New York Times*. https://www.nytimes.com/2020/04/22/us/politics/social-distancing-coronavirus.html

[15] Hatchett, R. J., Mecher, C. E., &Lipsitch, M., 2007. Public health interventions and epidemic intensity during the 1918 influenza pandemic. *Proceedings of the National Academy of Sciences of the United States of America, 104*(18), 7582–7587.

[16] Lewnard, J. A., & Lo, N. C., 2020. Scientific and ethical basis for social-distancing interventions against COVID- 19. *The Lancet Infectious Diseases*. https://doi.org/10.1016/S1473-3099(20)30190-0

[17] Maharaj, S. and Kleczkowski, A., 2012. Controlling epidemic spread by social distancing: Do it well or not at all. *BMC Public Health*, 12(1), p.679.

[18] Prem, K., Liu, Y., Russell, T.W., Kucharski, A.J., Eggo, R.M., Davies, N., Flasche, S., Clifford, S., Pearson, C.A., Munday, J.D. and Abbott, S., 2020. T*he effect of control strategies to reduce social mixing on outcomes of the COVID-19 epidemic in Wuhan, China: a modelling study.* The Lancet Public Health.

[19] Reluga, T.C., 2010. Game theory of social distancing in response to an epidemic. *PLoS computational biology*, 6(5).

[20] https://www.newsmedical.net/news/20200331/Eightstrains-of-coronavirus-afflicting-theworld.aspx

[21] Panchal, N., et al. 2020. The implications of COVID 19for Mental Health and Substance Use. Coronavirus (COVID-19). *Kaiser Family Foundation*, page 14.

[22] Ornell, F., et al. 2020. The COVID-19 pandemic and its impact on substance use: Implications for prevention and treatment. *Psychiatry research*, 289:113096.

[23] Qiu, J., et al. 2020. A nationwide survey of psychologicaldistress among Chinese people in the COVID-19 epidemic: implications and policy recommendations. *General Psychiatry*, 33(2):e100213.

[24] Nibudey, A., S, V. B. 2020. Preparing Hospitals in India for Covid-19 Pandemic. *International Journal of Research in Pharmaceutical Sciences*, 11(SPL1):333–341.

SECTION 2. POSITIVE AND NEGATIVE IMPACTS OF COVID-19

In: Impacts and Implications of COVID-19 ISBN: 978-1-53619-670-2
Editors: Anand Sharma et al.

Chapter 4

IMPACT AND CHALLENGES FOR THE INDIAN EDUCATION SYSTEM DUE TO THE COVID-19 PANDEMIC

Harish Sharma[1], Sourabh Singh Verma[2,*], Varuni Sharma[3] and Ajay Prasad[4]
[1]Department of CSE, School of Computing and IT,
Manipal University, Jaipur
[2]Department of CCE, School of Computing and IT,
Manipal University, Jaipur
[3]Department of Economics,
School of Humanities and Social Science,
Manipal University, Jaipur
[4]SoCS,University of Petroleum and Energy,
Dehradun, India

ABSTRACT

Coronavirus has upset the world in the years 2019-20. Every business and sector got affected due to the circumstances created

---

* Corresponding Author's E-mail: ssverma80@gmail.com.

by this epidemic. We should know the virology, epidemiology, and safeguards needed to take in this pandemic to understand its impact. Due to its highly contiguous nature, it is essential to save the next generation from its impact as much as possible. The education sector is one of the sectors, which have a huge number of youngsters evolved. Governments around the world have closed their educational institutes physically to stop its spread in public. But, this has raised the issue of hampering continuous education. Our article discussed the impacts, policies, capabilities, and responses taken by the Indian education sector during this pandemic lockdown. Also, we have examined the role of Information and Communications Technology (ICT) Tools and the Indian Government, which have enabled the students of Indian educational institutes to learn and continue their knowledge acquiring process.

Keywords: COVID-19, coronavirus, ICT, education, lockdown

INTRODUCTION

The spread of the Coronavirus pandemic has drastically unsettled various sectors in India. Education, aviation, travel, and hotel tourism industries are the most affected sectors among these. The education sector, which was considered the most profitable and secure sector in the last few years, now seems very tangled due to the everyday policy changes by the Government related to class conduction, examination guidelines, and fee uncertainty. It has created an exceptional test on the education sector.

In this chapter, we will discuss the major impact of the COVID-19 pandemic lockdown on the Indian education system and the measures taken by various educational Institutes and authorities to provide unprecedented services during this time of crisis.

ELEMENTARY KNOWLEDGE OF CORONA VIRUS

A coronavirus is an enormous group of infections, including some that cause the symptoms of the regular virus to some that cause significant sicknesses, for instance, the Severe Acute Respiratory

Syndrome (SARS) and the Middle East Respiratory Syndrome (MERS). COVID (nCoV) is another pandemic that has not been recognized in individuals previously. When scientists choose what COVID is, they give it a name (as under COVID-19, the disease-causing it is SARS-CoV-2).

Virology

The International Committee on Taxonomy of Virus (ICTV) has recognized Coronavirus as a severe acute respiratory syndrome coronavirus 2 (SARS-CoV-2) [1]. While on the other hand, ICTV found that the Middle East respiratory syndrome (MERS) virus is quite dissimilar with the COVID-19 [2, 3]. It appears that the primary source of the virus is bats, as the closest RNA sequence matches with the bat's coronaviruses. The way of transmission of the virus from bat to human is still unknown.

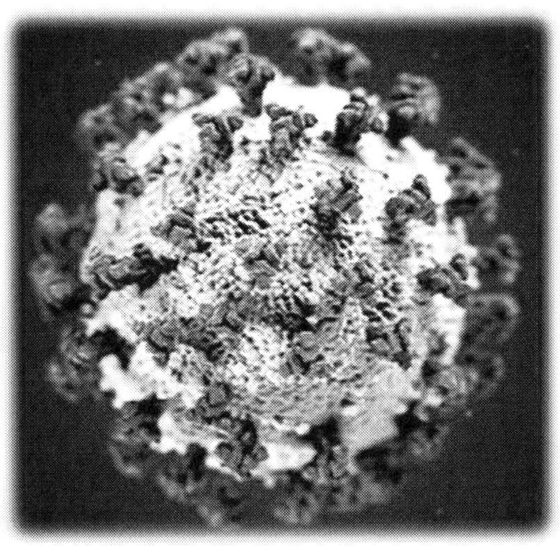

Figure 1. Coronavirus under the microscope.

Coronavirus is named like that because, under a microscope, it resembles a crown. The virus consists of protein spikes that surround the center of genetic material. Figure 1 shows coronavirus under a magnifying glass; it shows the genetic material at the center and shows various protein spikes. The presence of spikes gives it the looks of a crown. Corona is the Latin word for a "crown." The COVID-19 surged up and became noticeable when China informed about various instances of pneumonia due to unknown issues to the World Health Organization (WHO) on December 30, 2019. In China, it started at the Wuhan city of Hubei province. WHO confirms this by issuing a public release regarding the spread of the novel Coronavirus infection on January 09, 2020. Following this, in February 2020, the World Health Organization (WHO) named the 2019-nCOV epidemic COVID-19 [4].

Epidemiology

COVID-19 is similar to SARS and MERS as it can be transmitted from human to human through droplets, personal contacts, and virus contained objects. But, COVID-19 seems to be more deadly and spreadable as compare to other pneumonia. The epidemiology of the Coronavirus can be summarized as follows:

- Human to Human Transmission
- Period of infection
- Asymptotic or Symptotic Transmission
- Contamination
- Immunity
- Reinfection Risk

Epidemiologically it is determined that it can happen through short proximity contact; the main cause of the transmission from human to human is through droplets. It is found that droplets can travel around two meters. Therefore government bodies suggest maintaining social distance for at least six feet. Infection can also be possible by touching contaminated objects and possible cough, sneezes, and touch of an infected person.

The potential risk of the spread of infection from one person to another is at the initial stage of the disease; after ten days, the transmission is rare for a well immune person. Asymptotic or Symptotic Transmission is possible; that's why it is more difficult to stop transmission of the infection. The virus can also be present on the contaminated surfaces. Thus it can be transmitted to any individual by touching it, and then it can infect the person through mucous in the mouth, eyes, and nose. The duration of the virus's persistence on different types of surfaces is not exactly known, but it may survive till nine days on the surface like steel, etc. The reinfection of COVID-19 is quite low; nevertheless, to cite, a 33 years old person tested positive for the disease. But, reports say testing positive after the negative report does not always represent an infectious virus [5].

Clinical Presentation

Typically, Coronavirus symptoms are similar to other flu infections [6]. Nevertheless, in some of the cases, it may be asymptotic also. In the case of symptomatic patients, the symptoms may develop from mild to moderate levels. These symptoms may be present with respiratory uneasiness. Many researchers are doing their work to predict its impact on society [7, 8] and early diagnosis to reduce its harm [9].

Coronavirus is highly dangerous in some high-risk categories of people. WHO can categorize these as following [10]:

- Older People (greater than 60 years)
- People with diabetes
- Asthmatic persons, or people who are prone to lungs infections
- People suffering from heart issues
- hypertension
- Anyone suffering from some chronic disease like:
  - Cancer
  - Liver Disease
  - Kidney Disease

Symptoms of Coronavirus can be line-up as follows:

- Sore throat
- Muscular Fatigue
- Respiratory issues

- Fever
- Cough
- Breathing issues.

Besides of above symptoms, WHO identifies some emergency.

IMPACT OF COVID-19 LOCKDOWN ON INDIAN EDUCATION SECTOR

In India, lockdown due to the COVID-19 pandemic was started on March 22, 2020, to assess the country's preparation to safeguard against the corona spread. Then, it went till June 30, 2020, in different phases from Lockdown 1.0 to 5.0. In these lockdown phases, all the educational institutes remain closed and never got any relaxation. Thus, this lockdown created a huge impact on all educational institutes. The lockdown announcement just after the Holi festival vacation created a dilemma in the student and administrator as most of the institute was already closed for the short vacations. Most students could not carry the essential material for the study and ICT tools like computers and mobile to remain connected for online education.

Due to covid-19, various teaching and learning methodologies have emerged, and the same will continue in the future. Also, some suggestions for new methodologies and teaching-learning solutions will be discussed further.

The present study is focused on the following objectives:

- Present educational system before the pandemic and policies.
- Highlight the impact of Covid-19 on the Indian education sector.
- Enlighten various emerging challenges of Indian educational institutes for providing education during COVID-19 Pandemic lockdown.
- Role and emergence of various ICT-based solutions and MOOC is providing platforms.
- Discuss post-COVID-19 trends of various educational entities.

- Opportunities for new business and a new strategy for educational institutes.

Various reports of national and international agencies on the Covid-19 pandemic have been collected for our study. As it is not possible to go outside for data collection due to lockdown, information is collected from different authentic websites, journals, and e-contents relating to the impact of Covid-19 on the educational system in India.

More than 3 billion students and nearly 10 million employees working in the educational sector got affected by this lockdown policy in India. The COVID-19 pandemic taught the entire society the necessity of proper online learning, low-cost ICT tools and introduced virtual learning culture in Indian educational institutions. According to a UNICEF report, only 24% of Indians have internet connections to access e-education, and there is a large rural-urban divide that will widen the learning gap. Indian Education System can be broadly classified into three categories:

- Schools (Primary/Secondary and Government/Private)
- Colleges/Standalone Institutions (affiliated to some university)
- Universities and Deemed institutions (like IITs, Central Universities, Govt./Deemed/Private Universities, etc.)

Impact of COVID-19 Lockdown on School Education System

According to one of the reports by the Govt. of India portal (data.gov.in), there are nearly 15,22,346 schools in India in 2016-17. This includes Government, Private, Primary, Secondary, all kinds of schools providing education. Out of these, nearly 20% of schools have basic ICT infrastructure. Even this infrastructure is not able to support online education requirements like high-speed internet facilities.

There are very limited options available other than to shift to ICT-based Platforms from traditional classroom learning. This will be the biggest challenge as Indian education can't go online as only 8% of homes with a young generation below 18 years have computers with proper internet connection [11].

Most private schools cannot survive in this pandemic due to a lack of finance to support online education platforms. Various parent associations are asking reasons about the amount of fees schools are charging for the lockdown period. Private schools, which were considered one of the most profitable businesses in recent times, cannot satisfy the parents with any legitimate reply.

The most relevant reason can be the classification of school fees categories into tuition fees and sports fees, library fees, transport fees, and extra-curricular fees. In this present lockdown scenario, parents' arguments seem legitimate as schools are not providing sports, transport, and library facilities that they used to charge very high, although a different perspective from school administrators also needs to be discussed. Usually, schools plan their faculty's salary expenditure according to overall fees input. Still, due to lockdown and fund delay, schools will not provide salary to their staff which will deteriorate the situation even more. Proper fee re-structuring needs to be done by the private school such that both parents and faculties will get benefitted which will indirectly benefit the students.

Impact on Higher Education System

According to a survey report of the Ministry of Human Resource Development (MHRD), Government of India, there are nearly more than 1000 universities, 40,000 Colleges, and 12276 standalone institutions are working in India to provide higher education [12].

Many entrance tests (like IIT JEE, NEET, CUCET, etc.) for higher study got canceled, which created a great challenge in higher education. There is uncertainty about the admission process for new entrants for all the programs. The HEIs have started conducting orientation programs, induction meetings, and counseling classes with the help of different e-conferencing tools like Google Meet, Skype, YouTube live, Facebook live, WebEx, etc., to provide support services to the students. Student movement to other countries has been reduced, resulting in better admission in institutions available in India. Somehow, most of the institution has completed the final exams by online mode or by adjusting marks of midterm evaluations.

Researchers are not able to visit national and international labs and research centers. This harms the research activities, especially in the field where only limited laboratories have a particular environment for the respective research field. But, there are few positive implications too. Webinars and virtual summits have become normal these days. The researcher got more to improve their theoretical knowledge through these online activities.

There is no new recruitment in the Government sector in India, and recent pass-outs are under pressure of fearing withdrawal of job offers from corporate sectors because of the pandemic situation. Also, Private colleges and Private universities cannot pay full salary to their teaching and non-teaching staff due to delays in admission processes.

The Common Challenges for the Indian Education System in the COVID Lockdown Scenario

Under Mission Antyodaya, a national survey of villages was conducted by the Ministry of Rural Development in 2017-18[13]; this survey enlightened that 16% of India's households received 1-8 hours of electricity daily, 33% received 9-12 hours, and only 47% received more than 12 hours a day. While 24% Indians population has a smartphone, only 11% of families possess any type of computer, which includes desktop computers, laptops, notebooks, netbooks, palmtops, or tablets. Teachers and school administrators continue their communication with students through virtual lectures, Learning Management Systems (LMS), or portals like Massive Open Online Courses (MOOC) for teaching and curriculum activity. However, both teachers and students face unprecedented challenges in the absence of physical classrooms and proper digital infrastructure. Only moving classrooms to online mode would not mean effective remote learning. One-to-one interactions among peers and their mentor teacher are very important for proper learning. On any digital platform, student's learning and communication with others are largely dependent on the willingness of both teachers and students to accept the digital culture. In distance learning, the onus of culture is more on students, which requires discipline.

There are exceptional tasks for teachers also. Many Instructors are digitally unskilled; a large number of educators have never used an online environment for teaching purposes. Teaching a course online course in an ideal world requires more preparation, such as designing a lesson plan, an acquaintance of ICT Tools, and preparing teaching resources like presentation, audio, and video contents. This has posed new challenges for many teachers who are more apt toward traditional classroom teaching. Teachers are trying to improve their skills, but taking classes from home is a challenge for them because their family also needs to adopt this culture. Also, a large amount of data required to take online lectures during this period, so efficient use of that data is required. Schools and Other institutes are not providing any support to faculty for additional data charges for online classes.

Role of Indian Government Policies and Changes

Although the Central and State governments took many initiatives, there has not been enough expenditure on improvising the digital infrastructure for remote ICT-based learning during this pandemic. The Ministry of Human Resource Development budget [14] for digital e-learning was reduced to Rs 469 Crore in 2020-21 from Rs 604 crore in 2019-20.

Online classes regularly have a cost implication, too, as students have to abide by the cost of internet data services. There is no communication from governments on whether it will compensate students or provide free or subsidized data plans with the support of any telecom company like BSNL or Private vendor. In the present situation, many students, especially individuals whose families have lost incomes due to a lockdown-related employment loss, cannot afford such issues.

UGC & AICTE have released Guidelines on Examinations and Academic calendar given COVID-l9 pandemic and subsequent lockdown (UGC notice). But, as the government policies are kept changing, this calendar also keeps changing. All terminal examinations have been postponed and suggested commencement of classes from August 2020, which moved recently to November 2020.

Reopening schools for primary and middle classes is too risky, and if something happens to a child, the state government will be at the receiving end. While the state governments seem concerned that reopening of schools may trigger a spate of infections, the primary concern of parents is the safety of their children.

All citizens understand that it will be high risk to allow all students to join university and school. These places have long contact hours that will be responsible for the spread of a virus-like Corona. Indian Government & State's Governments are still working on a policy to allow these institutes to work normally. Meanwhile, we should appreciate the Government's earlier technical initiatives contributing during this pandemic time like SWYAM and NPTEL, etc. The MHRD-India and University Grants Commission (UGC) have launched many virtual platforms to learn to the home initiative in the last decade. These initiatives like online depositories, e-books, and other online teaching/learning materials, educational channels through Direct to Home TV, Radios for students are now looking very helpful for Indian students of various levels.

ICT Initiatives Taken for Education System in India

At the beginning of COVID-19, particular meeting apps like WebEx, Skype and Zoom become very popular as these were free-to-use applications; later, the Government has released an advisory to use Chinese applications with caution. As there are few rumors around, those applications like Zoom are sharing user data with the Chinese Government.

Although the Education sector does not come under sensitive sectors for national security, schools become more cautious about their data. Some of the digital initiatives of UGC & MHRD for higher education during COVID-19 are pointed as below:

Audio-Video Contents

Swayam Portal provides Massive Open Online Courses (MOOCs) with 140 universities-approved credit transfer features. Many universities are now becoming part of Swayam Local Chapters. The University Grant Commission (UGC) and AICTE have now issued a Credit transfer framework for online learning courses through their portal SWAYAM. Universities and institutions are permitted to assign 20% of the credits each semester for courses offered by SWAYAM in that particular semester.

For the student living in far places where internet facilities are possible, Swayam-Prabha provides high-quality educational programs through 32 DTH channels transmitting educational contents free of cost to all over India.

Gyandarshan (http://www.ignouonline.ac.in/gyandarshan/) is a web-based TV channel devoted to educational and developmental needs for Open and Distance Learner by Indira Gandhi Open University (IGNOU). A web-based TV channel devoted to the educational and developmental needs of the society

Digital Content (Journals and eBooks)

National Digital Library (https://ndl.iitkgp.ac.in/)project is sponsored by National Mission on Education through Information and Communication Technology (NMEICT) and arranged funding through the Ministry of Education. It is a repository with search and browse facilities and provides a host of facilities for the learner community. It provides interface support for the ten most commonly used Indian Languages. IIT, Kharagpur, develops it.

e-PG Pathshala (https://epgp.inflibnet.ac.in/) is for postgraduate students. Postgraduate students can access this platform for e-books, online courses, and study materials.

e-ShodhSindhu (https://ess.inflibnet.ac.in/) is a collection of e-journals and e-books on long-term access basis. It has 10,000+ e-journals, 164,300 E-Books in its database, and added to this 6 Lac e-books via National Digital Library (NDL). It provides facilities to use qualitative e-resources, including full textbooks, journals, bibliographic and real databases, to academic institutions at a nominal subscription rate.

Shodhganga (https://shodhganga.inflibnet.ac.in/) is a platform for collecting the Ph.D. dissertation of research students of Indian institutions and making it accessible to the whole scholarly community via open access. The depository has the facility to capture, index, and store, circulate and preserve Electronic Thesis and Dissertations submitted by the researcher's institution. UGC has made it compulsory for all Indian universities to provide a dissertation on this portal.

e-Adhyayan is an online platform that provides more than 700 e-books for under-graduation and post-graduation courses. All the e-Books are derived from e-PG Pathshala courses. It also facilitates a play-list of video content. A platform for e-books is the press book which is an open-source platform. It has been deployed and managed by the INFLIBINET center. Even Indian author can publish their book on this platform.

CBSE Podcast: CBSE launched a Podcast app, 'CBSE-Shiksha Vani,' available on the Play Store for Android phone users.

IIT Pal: For online coaching of IIT entrance exams, interested students can access lectures on physics, chemistry, mathematics, and biology on the official website of the National Testing Agency. [Website: https://nta.ac.in/LecturesContent]. By this platform, the student can prepare for the entrance exam from home.

UMANG mobile app: School students can move to e-learning on the Government's UMANG mobile app during a stay at home due to coronavirus outbreak lockdown. It contains more than 10 million e-books, audios, and videos on all subjects for primary and secondary school students.

This app provides the option of e-pathshala, where students can access books and study material of NCERT (National Council of Educational Research and Training).

Hand-on Learning Labs

One of the challenging tasks during this pandemic lockdown for engineering faculty was to conduct the laboratory for effective teaching and learning.

E-Yantra is a web platform that provides effective education across engineering colleges in India on Embedded Systems and Robotics in collaboration with IIT Bombay. The training for teachers and students is conveyed through workshops, where participants have learned the basics of embedded systems and programming. e-Yantra also helps colleges set up Robotics labs/clubs to make this activity a part of their routine teaching curriculum. More than 275 colleges across India have benefited from this particular initiative. All the projects and code are available on the e-Yantra website (www.e-yantra.org) as open-source content.

FOSSEE (Free/Libre and Open Source Software for Education) promotes open-source programming in instructive establishments (http://fossee.in). Through education data, such as audio tutorials, documentation, such as textbook companions, awareness programs, such as online conferences, training workshops, and Internships. Textbook Companion (TBC) is a collection of code for solved examples of standard textbooks.

Tools such as *Spoken Tutorial* (https://spoken-tutorial.org/) provides teaching and learning a particular FOSS (Free and Open Source Software) like Linux, Scilab, LaTeX, PHP & MySQL, Java, C/C++, LibreOffice, etc. using an easy Video tool - Spoken Tutorials.

Virtual Labs (http://www.vlab.co.in/) has developed web-enabled curriculum-based experiments designed for remote operation. This entryway gives far off admittance to Labs in different orders of Science and Engineering. These Virtual Labs oblige understudies at the undergrad level, the postgraduate level just as to investigate researchers.

Vidwan: is an extensive database that provides information in detail about experts to peers. It also provides vital information to prospective contributors, various funding agencies, researchers, and policymakers throughout the country.

The above Government initiatives benefit at a large scale to provide all levels of education and learning to Indian students at a very nominal cost. They only need an internet connection of adequate speed and a computing device for the access of content.

MEASURES TAKEN BY EDUCATIONAL INSTITUTES AND MOOC PLATFORMS

In addition to an initiative by the Government, various universities and institutes are initiating tie-ups with outside universities and online MOOC platform companies. MOOC platforms are reaching to its audience in a pandemic in the following ways:

- By providing course material and catalogs for campus students
- Informational courses for COVID-19
- Providing online free certifications

Coursera (www.coursera.org) provides various MOOC courses on nearly all disciplines, including engineering, arts, science, management, etc. It has a tie-up with most top institutes of the world. Although most of the free courses are not in-depth courses for the introductory level, they are enough. Coursera has emerged as a top MOOC platform by providing free access to all students and faculty to register licensed Institutes at nominal cost. Although this free access does not cover all the courses, most of the courses are available. Coursera allows you to enroll on its online platform that offers MOOCs, has increased rapidly, and it surged to 640% higher during lockdown comparing with last year enrolments; in this period, the numbers have grown from 1.6 to 10.3 million [15].

On April 24, Coursera stretched out a comparative proposal to governments, this time utilizing its Coursera Workforce Government Recovery activity. It would permit governments to give jobless specialists admittance to Coursera's index. Every legislature will get up to 50,000 licenses.

Edx (www.edx.org) provides more than 2500 courses from 140 institutes across the world. This includes Engineering, Computer, Humanities, Language, Business, Management, and Data Science. Although, we have seen some surge in the price of the courses during this pandemic time on this platform. It provides micro-bachelor, micro-master degrees also.

As a skilled developer, *Udemy* is an American-based massive open online course (MOOC) contributor. It provides support with 65+ languages around the globe.

Although most of the Platforms were majorly targeting college-going students, few Platform like Khan Academy is targeting the school-going young generation.

On the other hand, for MOOC suppliers like Coursera, edX, and FutureLearn, development didn't originate from campus to students, yet from social separating, strategies happening around the world.

By contrast, for MOOC providers like Coursera, edX, and FutureLearn, growth didn't come from campuses going online, but from social distancing, policies coming into effect worldwide.

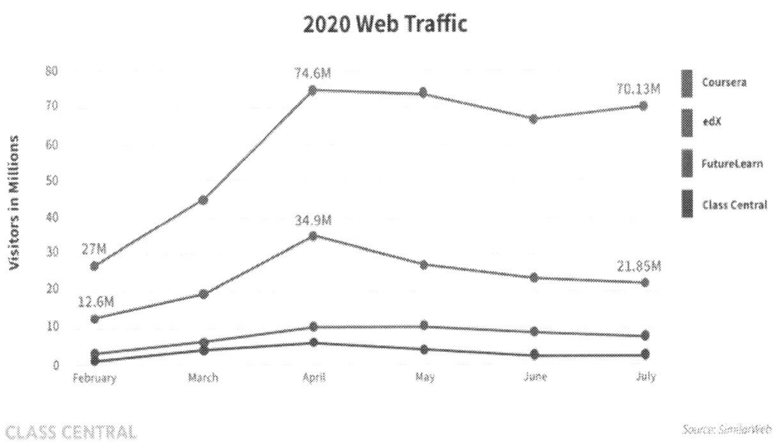

Figure 2. Web traffic change for top MOOC plate forms.

Table 1. Top ten subject by a number of followers pre & post-COVID-19 pandemic

Rank	Pre-Pandemic	Followers	Post-Pandemic	Followers
1	Computer Science	336k	Personal Development	167k
2	Programming	290k	Business	167k
3	Business	276k	Art & Design	117k
4	Personal Development	257k	Management & Leadership	115k
5	Management & Leadership	240k	Self-Improvement	113k
6	Data Science	235k	Humanities	112k
7	Artificial Intelligence	208k	Computer Science	110k
8	Information Technology	192k	Communication Skills	107k
9	Career Development	189k	Health & Medicine	106k
10	Entrepreneurship	188k	Foreign Language	106k

There are very few Indian platforms in this area. Still, after COVID, we have a very sudden rise in the start-up related to online education *UpGrade, Byju, Unacademy* is the Indian player who emerges as an Indian market leader for MOOC and Exam preparation. Whereas International platforms were targeting only international curriculum, Indian platform set their place by emerging as coaching platforms for Government Job, IAS, IES, GATE, and another national Competitive preparation platform.

During this pandemic lockdown period, it seems like now these MOOC platforms have become an essential part of education life. Indian universities and education institutes that were earlier very reluctant to accept these platforms and certifications are now allowing transferring credit for these courses. Even institutes are designing their own MOOCs.

POLICY SUGGESTIONS FOR THE NEW NORMAL: THE CONCLUSION

Firstly, AICTE must initiate the policy to fix the minimum number of computers in the institution so that appropriate usage of online classes and assignments may occur. Subsequently, the transparency in conducting the online assessment must be planned by conducting and promoting open book examination instead of the traditional patterns. For initial levels, assessment can be conducted using modes like quiz, test, walkthrough, etc. Subsequently, experiments, reports, models, projects, and self-evaluation can be done. These levels must be implemented on a step-by-step assessment basis. Like these, other tools may be invented or incorporated for assessments and assignments [16].

Many inevitable changes have been enforced upon society due to Covid-19. The opportunities created by the pandemic Covid-19 will lead towards a new tomorrow. Tomorrow will be something new than what we have expected earlier. The new way of learning will challenge the education sector to shift to a new pattern. Classroom lecture, mode assessment, and even attendance policies may need to change to respond to such shift in the expectation of new trends. Some of these expected new trends are list below [17, 18].

Increase in Demand for Open and Distance Learning

It will help students to learn at their pace and at a time of their choice. This will also augment Artificial Intelligence (AI) to help personalize a student's learning experience.

International Education Enrolment Will Reduce

Due to fewer travel options between countries, international travel will reduce. By Looking at the present poor health situation of the top countries like America, Italy, the UK, and France, the attraction toward foreign study will reduce. Our Indian national premium institutes like IIT,

NIT, IIIT, and Institutes of Eminence will get those students in This Scenario. So, they should take advantage of this situation.

Attendance Compulsion May Go Away

UGC, School Boards will not make attendance compulsory.

Multi Shift System in the Education System May Come

The face-to-face interaction in classroom teaching will take time to return, and almost surely, it will return with new norms such as a blended mode or changes in student-teacher ratio to maintain proper social distancing. This may result in the institute running multiple shifts or blended mode teaching methodology.

The Involvement of Technology Will Increase in Teaching and Learning

Augmented and virtual reality techniques can take book material to the next level to visualize experimental set-ups. AI and ML-based models can guide students by estimating their success rate to complete a course with satisfactory grades. AI system can also help students with special needs to get more equitable education, helping screen students with learning disabilities.

The Teacher Will Need to Update Themselves at a Higher Pace

Now, Teachers have to update themselves faster than earlier as students now have access to the most updated content.

The Teacher Will Become Mentor Rather Than an Academician

The role of teachers will be redefined. With the booming of Ed-Tech platforms to augment online learning, the role of a teacher from that of a 'knowledge-giver' will gradually shift to one of a 'facilitator' in the pedagogy system to help students become life-long learners.

Fall in Demand for Traditional Teaching Profession

If these pre-recorded MOOCs are so effective in teaching, then why is there a need to invest in expert faculty all over the country for a particular subject? This genuine query will certainly ignite in Education Institute owners that may lead to a decline in the number of faculty recruitment.

Shifting to Digital Operations of Education Institutes

Due to lockdown, schools and organizations have figured out how to move their authoritative and operational capacities to the digital world. Much has been transformed from online schedules, class and educator designations, and timetables to fund-related exchanges around charges and pay rates on secure computerized installment entryways; Indian schools have actively evolved and accepted the web. While most schools have just embraced the 'PC' for keeping records and building an information base of understudies and so forth, the lockdown enlivened digitization has driven them to make a total move, from tech upheld to tech-first tasks. Furthermore, this pattern is set uniquely to improve in a short duration.

Increase in Demand for Short Term Skilled Based Courses

To remain agile and relevant in the job market even after Covid-19, students must continuously upskill themselves with industry-ready courses. MOOCs are very helpful for professionals and those who already have some background knowledge about the subject and upgrade their skills. It is also helpful for self-motivated students who can invest time to find the answers to their queries while attending these courses. For a majority of the students, it may not be easy to connect with these lectures. However, online learning needs to go beyond MOOCs. They need to be based on interaction with the instructor [19].

Finally, we will come out of the COVID-19 pandemic sooner or later. It will give the Indian Education sector a kind of propulsion of changes that we need to take care of. Teachers, Schools, Institutes, and Universities need to change their attitude toward online education. Also, Classroom teaching cannot be disposable, but at the same time, using online ICT tools should be used to make the student comfortable in such lockdown situations and continue their education without interruption.

References

[1] Gorbalenya AE, et al., "Severe acute respiratory syndrome-related coronavirus: The species and its viruses – a statement of the Coronavirus Study Group," *Nature Microbiology*, 2020.

[2] Zhu N, Zhang D, Wang W, et al., "A Novel Coronavirus from Patients with Pneumonia in China, 2019," *The New England Journal of Medicine*, vol. 328, no. 8, p. 727, 2020.

[3] Lu R, Zhao X, Li J, et al., "Genomic characterization and epidemiology of 2019 novel coronavirus: implications for virus origins and receptor binding," *Lancet,* vol. 395, no. 10224, pp. 565-574, 2020.

[4] Centre of Disease Control & Prevention, *Information for Healthcare Professionals about Coronavirus (COVID-19),* CDC.gov, 25 AUG. 2020. [Online]. Available: https://www.cdc.gov/coronavirus/2019-nCoV/hcp/index.html. [Accessed SEPTEMBER 22 2020].

[5] Korean Centers for Disease Control and Prevention, *Findings from Investigation and analysis of re-positive cases,* CDC Korea, May 19, 2020. [Online]. Available: https://www.cdc.go.kr/board/board.es?mid=a30402000000&bid=0030. [Accessed September 20. 20].

[6] Public Health England, *COVID-19: epidemiology, virology, and clinical features,* Govt. of the UK, October 16 2020. [Online]. Available: https://www.gov.uk/government/publications/wuhan-novel-coronavirus-background-information/wuhan-novel-coronavirus-epidemiology-virology-and-clinical-features. [Accessed 24 Sep. 2020].

[7] Akshat Agrawal, Rajesh Arora, Ranjna Arora, Prateek Agrawal. (2021). Applications of Artificial Intelligence and Internet of Things for Detection and Future Directions to Fight Against COVID-19. In edited book on *Emerging Technologies for Battling Covid-19*, pp. 107-119, Springer.

[8] Prateek Agrawal, Vishu Madaan, Aditya Roy, Rajani Kumari & Harshal Deore. (2021). FOCOMO: Forecasting and monitoring the worldwide spread of COVID-19 using machine learning methods, *Journal of Interdisciplinary Mathematics*, pp. 1-25. doi: 10.1080/09720502.2021.1885812.

[9] V Madaan, A Roy, C Gupta, P Agrawal, A Sharma, C Bologa, R Prodan. (2021). XCOVNet: Chest X-ray Image Classification for COVID-19 Early Detection Using Convolutional Neural Networks. *New Generation Computing*, pp. 1-15, 2021. DOI: 10.1007/s00354-021-00121-7.

[10] World Health Organisation, "Coronavirus disease 2019 (COVID-19) Situation Report - 51," *WHO International*, [Online]. Available: https://www.who.int/docs/default-source/coronaviruse/situation-reports/20200311-sitrep-51-covid-19.pdf?sfvrsn=1ba62e57_10. [Accessed 14 March 2020].

[11] P. Kundu, "Scroll.in," *Scroll*, 05 May 2020. [Online]. Available: https://scroll.in/article/960939/indian-education-cant-go-online-only-8-of-homes-with-school-children-have-computer-with-net-link. [Accessed 01 Oct 2020].

[12] Department of Higher Education, "All Indian Survey on Higher Education," Ministry of Human Resource Development (MHRD), *Government of India*, Delhi, 2015-16.

[13] The Ministry of Rural Development, "Mission Antyodaya - a nationwide survey of villages," *Government of India*, Delhi, 2017-18.

[14] Ministry of human Resource Development, *Note on Demand for Grants*, Department of School Education and Literacy, India, 2020-21.

[15] D. Shah, "How Different MOOC Providers are Responding to the Pandemic," *The Report by Class Central*, May 02 2020. [Online]. Available: https://www.classcentral.com/report/mooc-providers-response-to-the-pandemic/. [Accessed September 25. 2020].

[16] K. P. Isaac, "When education goes digital," *The Hindu*, May 18 2020. [Online]. Available: https://www.thehindu.com/education/when-education-goes-digital/article31602533.ece. [Accessed 2020 Sep 14].

[17] *AI Business*, "Artificial intelligence in special education," March 21 2017. [Online]. Available: http://ai.business/2017/03/21/artificial-intelligence-in-special-education/ . [Accessed 14 Sep 2020].

[18] M. Lynch, "7 Ways That Artificial Intelligence Helps Students Learn," *The Edvocate,* May 01 2018. [Online]. Available: https://www.theedadvocate.org/7-ways-that-artificial-intelligence-helps-students-learn/ . [Accessed 10 Sep 2020].

[19] Chaturvedi, "Top 6 Ed-Tech trends in India post Covid-19," *India Today,* August 18 2020. [Online]. Available: https://www.indiatoday.in/education-today/featurephilia/story/top-6-ed-tech-trends-in-india-post-covid-19-1712071-2020-08-18. [Accessed 15 Sep. 2020].

In: Impacts and Implications of COVID-19 ISBN: 978-1-53619-670-2
Editors: Anand Sharma et al.

Chapter 5

IMPACT OF COVID-19 ON LIFESTYLE AND EDUCATION

***Vishu Madaan*[1], *Dileep Kumar P. Y. V. N*[1], *Prateek Agrawal*[1,2,*], *Anand Mohan*[3], *Charu Gupta*[4] and *Anand Sharma*[5]**

[1]Lovely Professional University, Punjab, India
[2]University of Klagenfurt, Austria
[3]P.G Department of Physics, C. M. Science College, L. N. Mithila University, Darbhanga, Bihar, India
[4]Bhagwan Parshuram Institute of Technology, New Delhi, India
[5]Mody University of Science and Technology, Laxmangarh, Rajasthan, India

ABSTRACT

COVID-19 or coronavirus or novel coronavirus, whatever the name is, becomes a buzz in the year 2020, which made the whole world prison and cost several lives. It disturbed the countries' economies and made it fall like a house of cards, and several people lost their jobs, income sources, and it has been a penalty for several

* Corresponding Author's E-mail: prateek061186@gmail.com.

students. Several organizations got affected, and some organizations shut down entirely where some of the organizations gained huge profits. This chapter performed a rigorous study to know how salaried people and students' lives are affected during this pandemic. We will also discuss what kind of significant changes came into the entire world's education system, how did this pandemic affect the jobs around the world, and how did it create opportunities for new businesses at the same time to grow.

1. Introduction

COVID-19 (Coronavirus or SARS-CoV-2) was originated from the food markets of Wuhan, China, in December 2019. It has now spread in almost the entire world and infected more than 100 million people in more than 190 countries. The World Health Organization (WHO) declared it a pandemic on March 11, 2020. COVID-19 pandemic has misbalanced and disrupted ecology and life cycle beyond repairs. In such a scenario, many challenges appear due to the inherent uncertainty involved with the disease outbreak. The outbreak of coronavirus disease 2019 (COVID-19) has created a global health crisis that has had a profound impact on the way we perceive our world and our everyday lives. COVID-19 is spreading across the world at an alarming speed.

Not only the rate of contagion and patterns of transmission threatens our sense of agency, but the safety measures put in place to contain the spread of the virus also require social distancing by refraining from doing what is inherently human, which is to find solace in the company of others. Within this context of physical threat, social and physical distancing, and public alarm, what has been (and can be) the role of the different stakeholders in our lives on individual, social and societal levels? It is an unprecedented crisis and calls for unprecedented measures. It affects human health, healthcare systems, global economy, business trades, manufacturing and service industries, transportation, etc. Nowadays, the government, policymakers, researchers, sociology professionals, healthcare and life science experts have constantly been working to deal with, deriving solutions, spreading positivity, and trying to protect humankind against COVID-19; there is also a significant focus on technological developments for improving the processes and mechanism for a better tomorrow. In the midst of all this, it was seen that the lifestyle of the people was affected. We are here highlighting few domains which have changed during the pandemic, and their impact will be seen on the human lifestyle for longer. Here in this chapter, we will discuss how the lifestyle of different persons changed and the difficulties or challenges, or opportunities created to rise during this pandemic.

2. Impact of the COVID-19 Pandemic on Employment

Containment measures have forced many businesses to close throughout the pandemic. In the developing world, many firms and workers operate in a large informal sector, often outside the scope of formal social protection, making them particularly vulnerable to restrictions imposed as part of the response to COVID-19. When we talk about employees, these are the people who suffered a lot during this pandemic. We can categorize employees into different kinds according to their area of work. There are a lot of industries/organizations in India, such as the Software/IT industry, Iron and Steel industry, Clothing industry, Construction industry, Automobile industry, which maintain massive labor forces; the ones who suffered job losses are primarily from the organization where the labors required heavily for everyday work. Simultaneously, there is a slight growth in job creation and that for the people above 50 years. People between the ages of 15 and 39 were most impacted by the Coronavirus (COVID-19) lockdown in India between April and July 2020 in terms of job loss. Those between 25 and 29 years old alone accounted for about 46 percent of all job losses. On the other hand, older Indians, close to nine million, gained jobs simultaneously [1]. We got the statistics of the job losses and the jobs gained in the previous year.

From Figure 1 statistics, we can clearly say that the pandemic hit the lives of people whose age is below 40 has been affected worst.

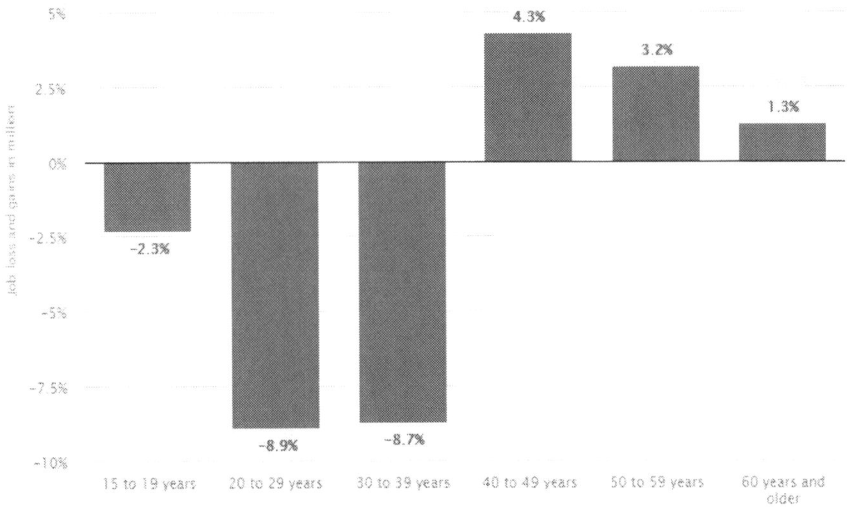

Source: https://www.statista.com/statistics/1125798/india-covid-19-impact-on-job-loss-by-age-group/

Figure 1. Jobs lost and gained in the Covid-19 era according to ages.

Most of the families in India depends on only one person who is working for his family and those are the people who suffered significant job losses ultimately the income issues raised and poverty increased and when it comes to the IT industry we can say there's significantly less percentage of employees lost their jobs but most of the employees got work from home facility to continue their work but here also there's significant changes came in their lifestyle increase of working hours and salary cuttings which ultimately leads to increase of stress levels which affected the mental health of the employees but here the IT industries seen huge profits than the previous years companies like TCS saw a huge profits last year and statistics for 2020-2021 yet to become so we can't post the statistics here but everybody knows the truth is each and every company is seeing huge profits compared to their previous years as they are extending the WFH facility further but ultimate loss is happening to the common man only organizations are seeing profits but not the employees . Moreover, based on these factors, we can say how their entire lifestyle got changed; we can discuss a small example over here about the WFH where the employees working from home are staying in their homes but are not able to lead an everyday life with their family from

Monday to Friday full-on work even for extra hours and the remaining days of Saturday and Sunday will be off to take rest. The mental work will make a man more tired than the physical work so as their week gets finished and next week is the same as continuing like that for months after the lockdown has been announced. Moreover, there is no such proof to say all of them face the issues, i.e., approximately “3 billion” service class people (except Defence and the healthcare sector) are compelled to work from home. It is affecting their mental health negatively, and some of them may be feeling isolated. The main thing is the home distractions because if you are staying at home, you have to take part in most of your household works, whatever it may be like bringing groceries and taking care of your children and your parents and especially the younger ones they do not know about what we are doing so they might cause some interruptions to your work likewise there are so many distractions one need to face when he is pushed to WFH. One of the essential affecting things is poor broadband speeds, i.e., the internet facilities. India is still a developing country where people do not have good network connections in many locations; this leads them to allocate more time to finish. Moreover, if we talk about the advantages of WFH, the advantages over 90% are for the organizations only. There are significantly fewer advantages to the employee like flexibility in working, and you stay with your family which is not possible in the standard times as many people have to go out of their states to work and you have to take care of your well being and health, but if you stay in home your family will take care of that yes we can say these are some of the advantages an employee can have.

See, in this world, almost everything got affected due to the novel Coronavirus, which emerged as the pandemic situation throughout the world, which originated from China, so let us see some of the areas where job losses occurred.

1. Due to coronavirus Air India withdraws job offers of nearly 180 cabin crew who finished their training and are ready to join the service.
2. In the United States alone, 6.6 million people applied for unemployment benefits in a single week in March 2020.

3. Infosys freezes its hikes and promotion to the existing staff in order to honor the job offers issued by the company.
4. Nearly 20 lakh job losses occurred in the transportation community, which includes cars, buses, and taxis.
5. In India, the jobless rate has increased to 23% more due to covid-19.
6. UK postal operator Royal Mail announced that it is going to cut nearly 2000 jobs.
7. The aviation giant Boeing slashed nearly 1200 jobs due to air travel and no demand for passenger jets.
8. Australia's Qantas airlines dropped 6000 employees due to the outbreak of the Novel Coronavirus.
9. Uber lays off number of employees, and even the CTO of the company stepped down.
10. The United Kingdom car sector axed 2000 employees due to decrease in the sales due to coronavirus fears.
11. Berger has not issued even a single job offer in the last year as the outbreak of Coronavirus.
12. Automobile giant industries like Bajaj auto, Tvs Motors, Tata motors axed the salaries to their employees.
13. Johnson Matthey, halves the largest producer of autocatalyst in Europe, laid down 2500 jobs.

So there are so many other jobs over there which has been lost due to this pandemic it will take nearly 10-20 papers more if we list all, so we listed some of them here, but we can access all the information from a place so here is the link for that place which helps you to find all the info [https://www.bls.gov/ces/publications/highlights/2020/current-employment-statistics-highlights-12-2020.pdf] in this link, they provided details of every industry-related employees hiring and laying off employees in a particular year up to the last ten years. From Figure 2, it is clarified that how many are going to become jobless in the COVID era is just a claim made by some statisticians but not done in real even the mark went nearly close as per the claims.

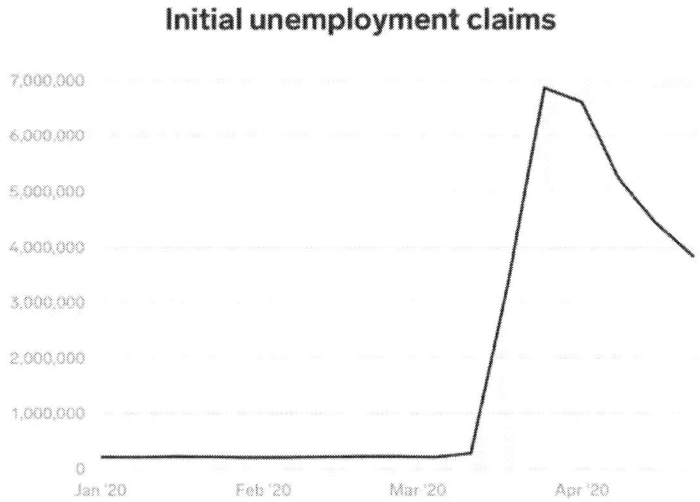

Source: US Employment and Training Administration via FRED. Business Insider.

Figure 2. Unemployment claims Due to pandemic in the initial stage.

3. Impact Of The COVID-19 Pandemic on the Education System and Students

As earlier, we discussed employees' lives, how their daily routines got changed and how it affected them in leading their life as, like employees, the students also got affected majorly by this Covid-19 pandemic. Their daily routine becomes like waking up, taking meals, attending online classes completing the assignments and following the same routine theme the next day. In India, when it comes to online education, several students stopped listening to the classes they turn on, and they do some other works, and some students even committed suicides because they do not have the equipment to attend the online classes.

1. Several incidents happened like that; we will mention a few of them here.This incident happened in Kerala Malappuram district, a young girl in Malappuram district despaired. She had neither a TV nor a smartphone. In the afternoon, the Class 10 student

went missing from her house. Her charred body was found from a deserted spot near her home around 3.30 pm. The girl was a bright student but set herself on fire as the government provided the classes through an online television (TV) channel, but her father, a daily wager, had no money to either repair the TV or buy a smartphone for her. There was no work for him to earn money because of this pandemic which snatched the life of his 14 years old daughter "Devika Balakrishnan". After this incident, a report came that an estimated 2.5 lakh students in the state do not have access to either a TV or devices that can access the Internet.

2. In another incident at Tamilnadu Theni district, a class 11th student, "Vikrapandi," died by suicide after failing to cope with the pressure of online lessons. He committed suicide because he could not understand online classes clearly and got scared that he would not fulfill their parents' dream of educating him [6].
3. Another incident was from Gujarat Rajkot, where a 12 years old "Kushi" hanged herself to death as she could not manage all the stress she was dealing with in the online classes.
4. In another incident, a B.sc second-year student, "Nithyashree" from Ulunderpet, Tamilnadu, committed suicide after facing many arguments with her two sisters over sharing the mobile phone to attend the classes because the three had to share the single smartphone for the online classes.

While here we are not saying because of online classes, only the suicides happened, but it also led them to commit death. It sickened them mentally, and some felt that they are alone, and the term "online classes" is a new concept and has not been that effective as the students have physical education for more than years. Suddenly these online classes are felt new and trouble for them and created a mental illness and fear in several students whether they will be able to study well or their studies going not or adequately into so many confusions and not having proper mentoring or guidance from elders made them feel like that there is nothing left for them and killing themselves. Their bright future became a way for the above. We highlighted a very few incidents which came in the news, but there are many similar incidents where the students died, and nobody knows, so it created a somewhat lousy impact on the students.

On the other side, the students having all facilities have improved their knowledge and learned so many new things as they got precious time freely to explore a lot. As we know, a coin has two sides; everything has positive impacts and negative impacts.

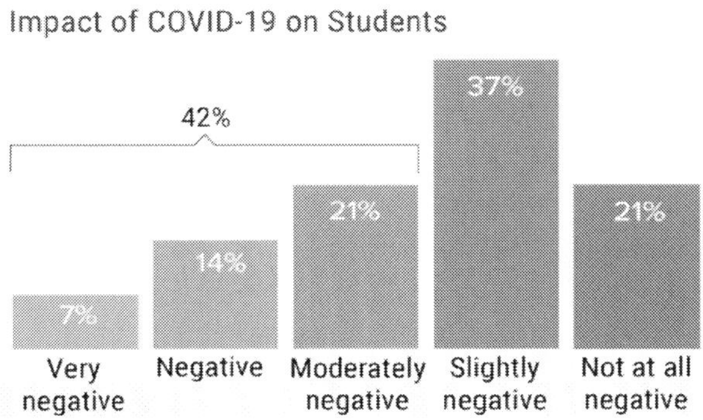

Source: https://www.google.com/url?sa=i&url=https%3A%2F%2Fwww.medscape.com%2Fslideshow%2F2020-medical-student-report-6013282.

Figure 3. Impact of covid-19 on students.

Figure 3, the explanation given to us is about the report taken from medical students on how their education system and daily life were affected by the pandemic.

We saw considerable changes in the educational system throughout the world during this pandemic. Exams got canceled due to the fear of COVID-19, and academic year schedules were changed. Entire education got transformed to online as like some online courses where the government offered the classes through the television channels there is two software we have to talk about which played a vital role in conducting online classes "Google Meet and Microsoft Teams". There is another one called ZOOM which got the rejection after some days due to security reasons while Microsoft Teams registered a 50% jump in numbers with 115 million daily active users at the end of October 2020, but zoom and google meet became the top downloaded apps of the year which is published in AppAnnies latest report.

When it comes to Google-meet, its day-over-day growth surpasses 60 percent. According to google, Google Meet's current usage has been increased to 30 times what it was in the starting month of the year, i.e., January 2020. More than 3 million connected users on Google meet every day and spent more than 3 billion minutes together, which we can say as 3,800 years of closed meetings every day was conducted in a single day in 2020. Google-meet Google's video conferencing product has surpassed 50 million subscribers on the play store as work from home numbers increased due to pandemic; since January, Google-meet daily usage has grown by three times than normal usage according to Google [10].

Nevertheless, whatever or how many users used have increased for both Google-meet and Microsoft teams; tech analysts described 2020 as the year of zoom. From 10 million connected users to 300 million users between December 2019 to April 2020 produced huge profits to Zoom in the third quartile of the financial year of 2020 has jumped by 36% year-over-year to $777.2 million. By the time both Google-meet and Microsoft teams were allowed for pay and use, the Zoom was free to use, which made it see everything from wedding to family meeting and even funeral attendings all went online. Many other virtual events took place in Zoom but after that due to its weak security everyone stopped using it and shifted towards Teams of Microsoft and Google Meet platforms.

When it comes to conduct classes online, the Universities and engineering colleges opt Google-meet and Microsoft teams in education sector. Some universities developed their software to provide high-quality online classes facility to their students, for example, Lovely Professional University, Phagwara, Punjab, India developed its platform: MyClass platform, to conduct online classes which are having several features including time table of classes every day and the recording of the classes will be stored according to the date of the class happened, incase if the students miss the class they can recess it, and some other features are there in it. Likewise, some other universities are also using their teaching platforms. In India alone, 32 crore college students are affected due to this pandemic incorporating faculties and facilities according to the report of UNESCO; and another major issue is the broadband speed. It is okay with Tier-2 and Tier-3 cities, but what about Tier-1. No doubt at all that E-learning will rise at a rapid pace, and companies like Udemy are going to help in this new education revolution.

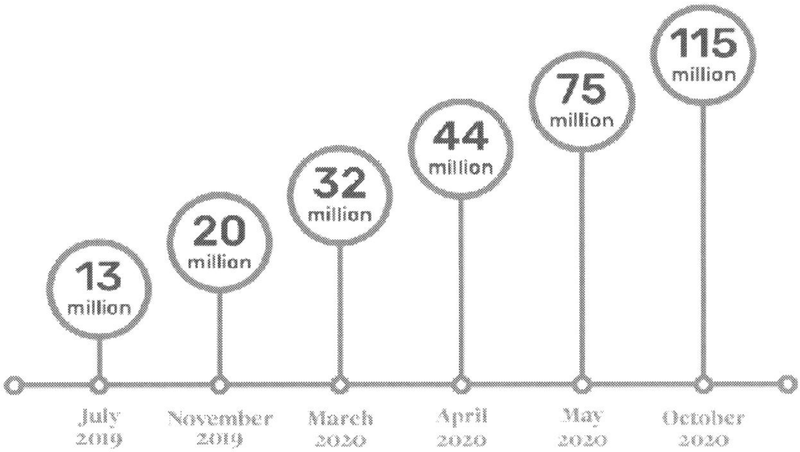

Source: https://tomtalks.blog/2020/12/microsoft-teams-statistics/

Figure 4. Increased users for Microsoft teams in millions due to online education.

Now let us see the statistics of the Zoom App, which emerged as the leading platform for online meetings and how it utilized the pandemic to grow its market, and how it helped a lot of students and lots of organizations throughout the world.

When the lockdowns started, Zoom lifted the limits for the accessible version of its software in China and educators in many countries, including the UK, helping to drive its popularity.

From Figure 4 and 5, we can see how the online meeting platforms got huge profits and even the growth of its industry, creating many opportunities for new companies, which helps the people stay more effective in this online world.

In Figure 6, it is mentioned that Close to a billion people are still locked down after the coronavirus outbreak brought the life around the world to a virtual standstill. The pandemic is expected to have enormous economic consequences, and it is also having a devastating impact on global education. According to the latest figures released by UNESCO, some 1.3 billion learners around the world were not able to attend school or university as of March 23, 2020 [12].

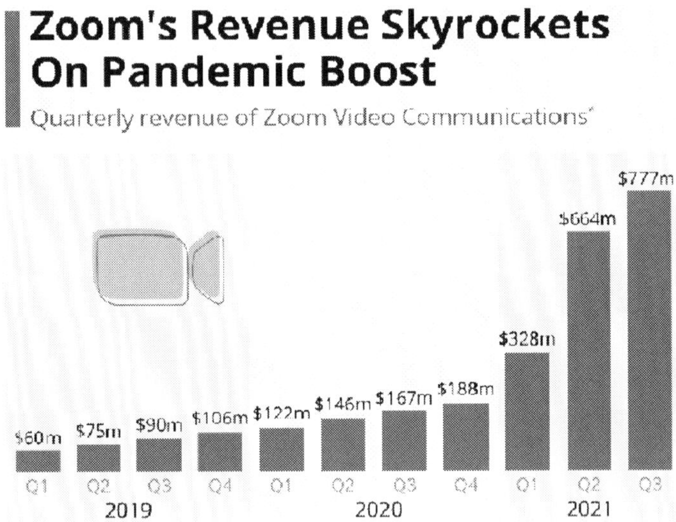

Source: https://www.statista.com/chart/21906/zoom-revenue/
* Zoom's fiscal year 2021 ends January 31, 2021.

Figure 5. Zoom revenue in millions due to covid-19.

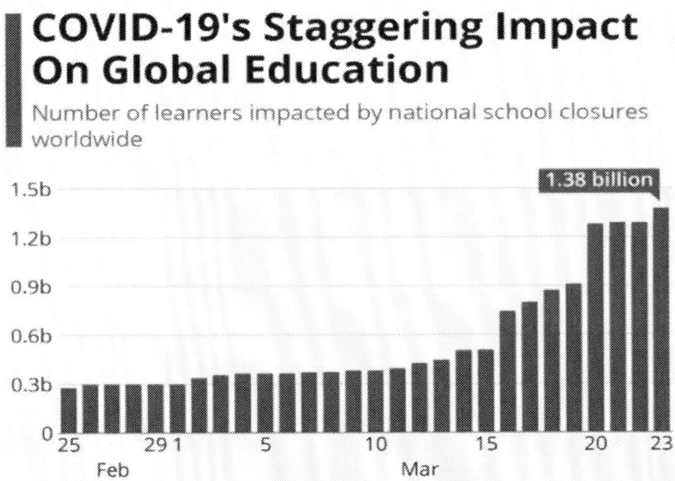

Figures refer to learners enrolled at pre-primary, primary, lower-secondary, and upper-secondary levels of education, as well as at tertiary education levels.

Figure 6. Affected students due to Coronavirus in billions.

Furthermore, if you want to study the new education policy introduced and supported by the central cabinet of India, go to the official website of the education ministry or just search on the Internet about the new education policy introduced by the central government of India. We see that number of children are affected by this COVID-19 due to staying out of their classroom and missed so much to get in school. There are 1.38 billion learners impacted by the national school closure worldwide, including all tiers of education. However, online education was not introduced in 2020. It has been out there for years. Would you believe online education is there for 170 years companies like Coursera, EDX, ByJus, Udemy, SkillShare, LinkedIn Learning, etc., are there in the online education market for years, but online learning came into focus because of this pandemic? In many economically weaker countries which are not digitized, online education is challenging. A coin has two sides; online education also has its pros and cons. The students having good broadband speed and the gadgets to access the online content are pretty satisfied with this system, while the students without these resources struggled to participate in online learning, and some even ended their lives due to the stress and pressure created by this system. Several institutions collect the same fee they are charging on regular days, even for this online teaching, and the faculty who is teaching the students are also not getting full salary in some areas. Many parents who lost their earning sources during the pandemic could hardly arrange their wards' school/college fees. Some Indian states called off the exams to promote the students for higher secondary education due to COVID-19 but got them promoted to the next class, somehow compromises the certificate value, unlike the previous years' students. So the changes which happened for the education system benefited some startups and organizations heavily. So one thing got clarified the online system got benefited due to this pandemic, and this pandemic crippled the offline system.

4. Impact of the COVID-19 Pandemic on E-Commerce

COVID-19 pandemic affected the Economy and GDP of several countries, and it also affected several startups and businesses all over the world badly. However, it does not apply to all as we can see tremendous growth seen by some companies like e-Commerce sites and online retailers compared to their previous years. Now, several companies and small businesses are shifted online. There is a massive increase in digital payment gateways like Phonepe, Google-pay, Paytm, etc.

The COVID pandemic shifted e-commerce in 2020, maybe more than any other time in history. Traditional retail sales have declined, but e-commerce has seen a 129% year-over-year growth in US and Canadian orders as of April 21, with an impressive 146% growth in all online retail orders [8].

People are shifting buying habits across the world, and the lockdown has even hit boomers by forcing them to shop online – some for the first time. COVID has accelerated the e-commerce industry's growth, and more businesses are joining the e-commerce business revolution than ever before [8].

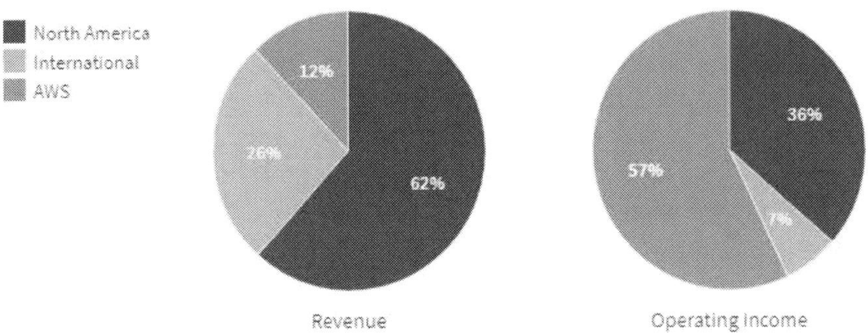

Source:https://www.investopedia.com/how-amazon-makes-money4587523s

Figure 7. Segmentation breakdown of amazon Income sources.

The Indian online E-commerce giants like Amazon and Flipkart have other businesses like Amazon web services, phone pay, amazon pay, amazon prime, etc. Now we will talk about the Amazon India growth. It has revenue loss in the year 2020. Year 2020 was not a bad year for amazon as they have seen 43% growth in their revenue compared to 2019 their revenue increased from INR 7,593.5 Cr to INR 10,847.6 Cr. However, they have faced a whopping loss of INR 5849.2 Cr as they invested 16,877.1 Cr for the financial year 2020 compared to 2019 they invested 13,463.1 Cr, but in 2020 the expenses also become high when compared to 2019 they saw nearly 25% increase in expenses, and we all know how famous Amazon is when it comes to marketing they spent up to 2330.7 Cr for Advertising only.

Figure 7 shows the clear segmentation breakdown of amazon's income sources from which areas it is earning its profits and its spendings on those particular areas.

India's most prominent e-commerce players by market share, Amazon and Flipkart, have together raked in $3.5 billion (about Rs 26,000 crore) during the first four days of their flagship festive season sales events, multiple brands and industry analysts told ET, with both the online marketplaces on track to meet expectations for the entire seven-day period [3].

Well, Amazon does not get backed by any large or small scale companies, but Flipkart got all the support it needed which Walmart backs, and it is having it is fashion retail company Myntra and saw a growth of 12% in it is revenue of INR 34,610 Cr, and it cuts it is losses by 18% compared to the previous year where it is retail subsidiary Myntra cuts it losses by 25% and saw a revenue of INR 4,262 Cr. In the previous year 2018-19, it has a revenue of 30,931 Cr and the net loss during this year was 3,835 Cr whereas, in 2020, it was reduced to 18% in number 3,150 Cr, the main income source for Flipkart is wholesale products and commissions from vendors to facilitate for sales of products and advertising like these, and yes Flipkart also do advertising equally to amazon as they both are the online rivals. For the financial year of 2020, Flipkart saw an 8.6% increase in its expenses. In an interview, Flipkart officials said that their main revenue-generating sources are E-commerce, Information technology-Enabled services, marketplace, and related support services. Moreover, another big news is that they included companies like Phonepe and Jabong into their organization; as we all know, Walmart nearly purchased 77 percent shares in Flipkart to become more powerful in the online retailers and sellers industry.

Some other companies like Snapdeal, Paytm mall, etc., are not that much popular, and even their revenue is less than 1000 Cr. On Snapdeal, the home products category selling kitchen appliances, linen, home décor, and LED lights grew 30% over last year, the value-focused e-commerce platform said, overtaking fashion, traditionally the top-performer during the sales period [3]. A company named AJIO, backed by reliance industries giving a tough competition to Myntra as it is not known to several people, there is an online fashion retailer named AJIO. However, the company's sales have grown this year in huge numbers and become a major competitor for Myntra, where AJIO achieved a four-times growth till October 2020, which surpasses well-known companies like Snapdeal, Tata Cliq, Koovs, etc. While the website visits of Ajio are more than Myntra, they have not reached the app downloads of Myntra yet. Let us see some statistics over here about the Comparison of Ajio and Myntra. The e-fashion market statistics include the monthly visits for every platform and the monthly downloads of each, and the average usage duration per day and month for all of the platforms are represented here.

	AJIO	MYNTRA	KOOVS	snapdeal	TATA CLiQ
Average monthly visits	23.5 mn	21.1 mn	0.6 mn	13.7 mn	5.7 mn
Average visit duration	5 min 24 sec	8 min 33 sec	2 min 10 sec	10 min 08 sec	19 min 07 sec

Source: https://www.businessinsider.in/business/ecommerce/news/reliance-backed-ajio-is-riding-on-the-indian-e-commerce-wave-poses-tough-competition-to-myntra/articleshow/78996579.cms.

Figure 8. Monthly traffic of e-fashion websites in the covid-19 period.

Currently, the penetration of online shopping at 4% will go up to 10 - 15% over the next 3 to 5 years. The fashion market in India is currently estimated at $70Bn, of which only 25% is organized retail. E-commerce is a key channel for fashion, and the online fashion market is projected to grow 3.5X from $4Bn to reach $14Bn by 2020 [7].

Figure 9 showing AJIO's latest numbers that it is leveling up to Myntra while moving fast ahead of other competitors like Tata Cliq, Snapdeal, and Koovs. While AJIO's website visits are higher than Myntra, it lags in app downloads and users [13].

	AJIO	MYNTRA	KOOVS	snapdeal	TATA CLiQ
Monthly downloads	5.6 mn	8.4 mn	0.2 mn	2.9 mn	2.1 mn
Daily active users	0.6 mn	2.3 mn	0.07 mn	0.92 mn	0.2 mn

Source: https://www.businessinsider.in/business/ecommerce/news/reliance-backed-ajio-is-riding-on-the-indian-e-commerce-wave-poses-tough-competition-to-myntra/articleshow/78996579.cms.

Figure 9. Monthly downloads of e-fashion applications in 2020.

AJIO scaled new highs with 4x growth in orders from pre-COVID levels. Its quarterly revenue run rate is now equivalent to full last year's revenue," said Reliance during its earnings results on October 30 [13].

5. Rise of the E-Pharmacy in the Digital Era

Everybody is aware of the word "pharmacy," even before the covid-19 attack, but due to increased sales of smartphones and online usage, pharmacy has entered into the digital market and makes a good amount of profits and fulfilling customers' requirements. When it comes to the digital drug (medicine) market, we got Netmeds, 1mg, Pharmeasy; these three are ruling the digital healthcare world. They saw huge profits in 2020 rather than the physical medicine shops people are shifting towards the online to save their time to reduce the contagion. So it worked well for them, and even the bigheads of e-commerce are trying to lay their foot into this drug market. Amazon is in talks with Apollo Pharmacy to invest 100 million dollars, while the reliance groups took a majority stake in the Netmeds online pharmaceutical company in approximately 80 million USD. Tata group is also in a queue to acquire a majority stake of another online pharma company, "1mg".

Another online pharma retailer company, the Pharmeasy, is already backed by several companies from different countries like Singapore's "Temasek holding","Lgt group", the CDPQ of Canada and Tpg of America, is ready to invest 1.2 billion dollars, and Nespers of Africa is ready to invest 100 million dollars in Pharmeasy. These deals came into talks when these online pharmacy companies saw huge growth within the few months after the lockdown was announced.

Before the pandemic, the e-pharmacy market had hardly 3 million users, while after the pandemic, it has grown to 6 more million new customers as per the FICCI report. Moreover, the big news is that the Indian online pharmacy market will rise to a 2.7 billion$ market by 2023, which is now a 360$ market.

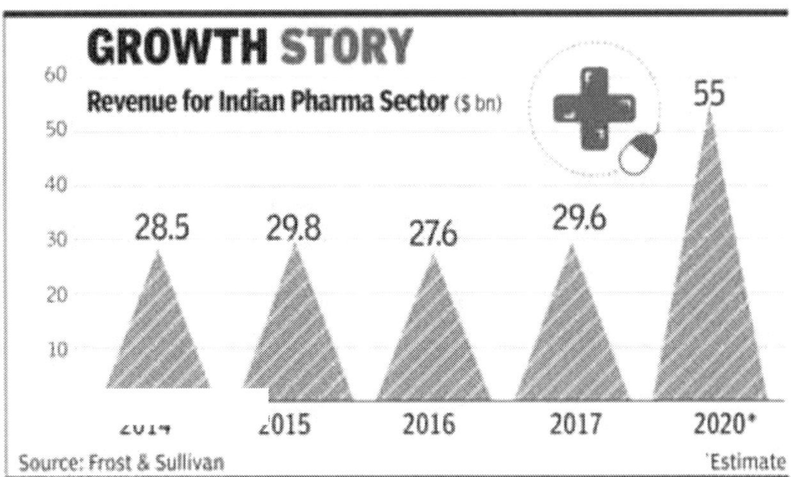

Source: Frost & Sullivan.

Figure 10. Growth of Indian pharma industry.

According to their ranges High, Low, Medium, in the above figures 10 and 11 it is clearly shown that the areas that have seen a rise in e-pharmacy in the world market. In the future, it will become a trend in the online business world which will create an impact on the online market. The e-pharmacy market is moderately competitive, with few players currently dominating the market. The key market players of the studied market comprise CVS Health Corporation, Albertsons Companies, Inc., ALTO, Axelia Solutions (Pharmeasy), among others [5].

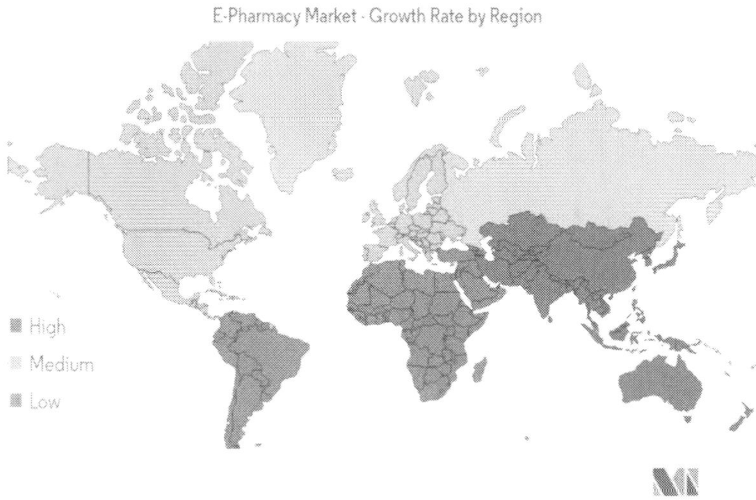

Source: Mordor Intelligence.

Figure 11. Rise of E-pharmacy in the world according to range.

6. Digital Buyers

In India since 2014, there is a continuous growth in digital buyers and online shopping where the number of online retailers is increasing. Users are getting attracted to shop online from different companies due to big discounts and offers, especially electronic goods. Household machines to fashion marketing, everything went online after seeing such a huge growth in users year to year. The statistics of users' growth from 2014 to 2020 in India are shown in Figure 12.

Figure 12 shows the paradigm shift of users from offline shopping to online shopping over the last few years. The main reason behind this growth is the excessive usage of mobile phones. Nowadays, everybody is using a smartphone, and companies like Jio made internet charges low. Ultimately, the remaining networks also made their fare low, so every user is accessing the Internet. Moreover, we can see the statistics of the average spendings of a person on the e-commerce stores monthly from Figure 13.

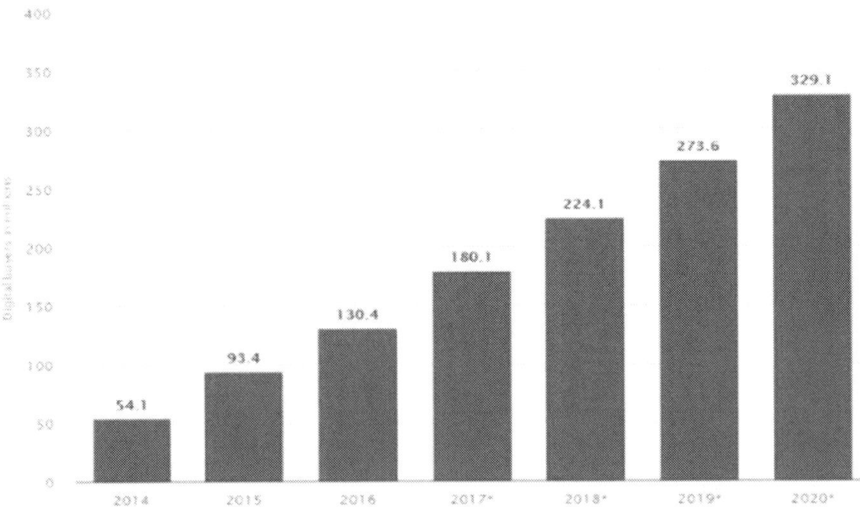

Source: https://www.statista.com/statistics/251666/number-of-digital-buyers-worldwide/

Figure 12. No. of digital buyers in India since 2014.

As we have the limited data and the data yet to come, we can see limited results only here, and we can see how the online shopping companies making profits in the particular season by giving offers we call festive offers and surprisingly the festive sales in 2020 saw a huge rise compared to its previous years.

Moreover, even the number of digital shoppers will increase at a particular time, called festive seasons. Companies like Flipkart, Amazon, Snapdeal target festival seasons and offer attractive offers to the customers to increase their sell. When it is up to e-fashion, there are always offers that drag the user's attention by showcasing a wide range of fashion clothes that many users will not find in their locality. Let us see the increasing rate of online shoppers in 2020 compared to the previous two years, shown Figure 14.

So there is a loss for the business which is not online. Almost all online businesses end up as profitable, and we saw a major shift towards online business. Several businesses have turned online and started providing their services. While let us talk about some of the businesses which saw losses and even some of them ended their business like Gym centers, Malls, Movie Theaters, Entertainment Parks, Hotels like such companies faced losses during this pandemic.

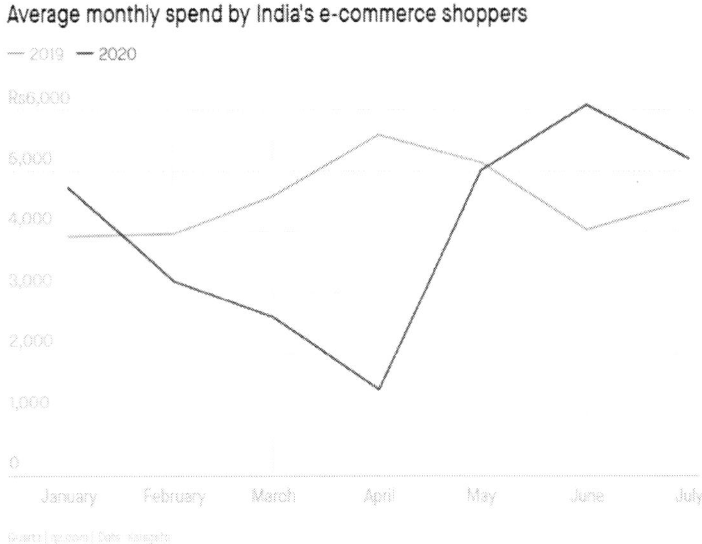

Source: https: seekingalpha.com/4377492-opportunities-in-india-e-commerce.

Figure 13. Monthly spendings of Indian online shoppers.

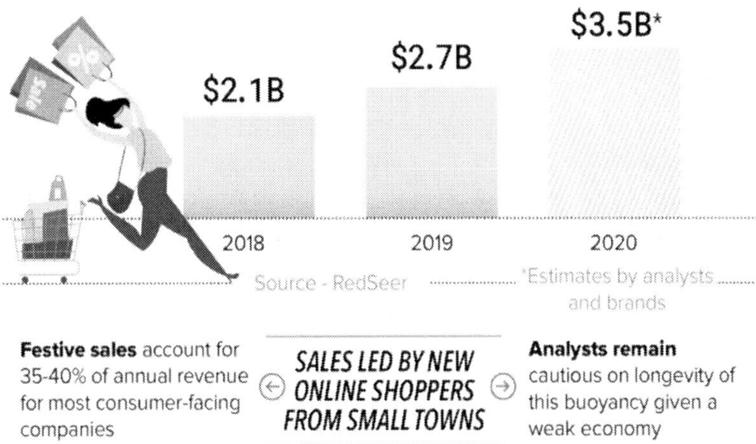

Figure 14. Increase in sales of e-commerce during festive seasons.

Well, now let us take a look towards the online Grocery shopping like Amazon and Flipkart here also got BigBasket and Grofers are the rivals in the online grocery market, a simple example of how fast the online grocery market is evolving when compared to the E-commerce saw only 6% growth compared to its previous year. In contrast, online grocery industry saw nearly 76% growth see how much difference is there in the numbers. Per day BigBasket delivers nearly 3 Lakh orders. Can you imagine how many, before the pandemic, there were hard up to 1500 deliveries per day? E-commerce got a market value of 33.5 billion dollars which was increased to 35.1 billion dollars, whereas the online grocery market has a value of 1.7 billion dollars which was increased to 3 billion dollars. The market value is less when compared to e-commerce, but their growth is increasing faster than e-commerce.

So the ones who turned their businesses online have survived the pandemic while the others suffered now. We can say 2020 is not a bad year for all and not a good year for all, and when it comes to OTT platforms, we got several like Netflix, Amazon Prime, Disney Hotstar, etc., which saw profits in this year as the Movie theaters remain closed, so it is bad for one which turned to be good for another.

CONCLUSION

Here we conclude that nothing is bad in the world if you look deep into it; whatever happens, it creates both negative and positive impacts. As corona also leads to both negative and positive impacts on the living beings of this world. We have to accept that COVID-19 created negative impacts among the people and gave opportunities to some Sectors. We can say that it is a warning and a lesson to the people to get prepared for any situation that can lead to the extinction of the human race and change the lifestyle into a different kind.

REFERENCES

[1] Statista. 2021. *India: COVID-19 impact on jobs by age group 2020 | Statista*. [online] Available at: <https://www.statista.com/

statistics/1125798/india-covid-19-impact-on-job-loss-by-age-group/> [Accessed 17 February 2021].

[2] Statista. 2021. *India - estimated quarterly GDP impact by coronavirus 2021 | Statista*. [online] Available at: <https://www.statista.com/statistics/1103120/india-estimated-impact-on-gdp-growth-by-coronavirus-epidemic/> [Accessed 17 February 2021].

[3] Shrivastava, A. and Mukherjee, W., 2021. *Amazon, Flipkart combined festive sales hit $3.5 billion in just four days*. [online] The Economic Times. Available at: <https://economictimes.indiatimes.com/tech/technology/ecomm-festive-sales-hit-3-5-billion/articleshow/78779243.cms?from=mdr> [Accessed 17 February 2021].

[4] Sleeknote. 2021. *15 Eye-Opening Online Shopping Statistics for 2020*. [online] Available at: <https://sleeknote.com/blog/online-shopping-statistics> [Accessed 17 February 2021].

[5] "E-Pharmacy Market I Growth, Trends, COVID-19 Impact, and Forecasts (2021 - 2026)." *Home | Mordor Intelligence*, https://www.mordorintelligence.com/industry-reports/epharmacy-market. Accessed February 18 February 18, 2021.

[6] Nath, Akshaya. "Tamil Nadu: Unable to Handle Stress of Online Classes, Student Dies by Suicide - India News." *India Today*, India Today, September 3, 2020, https://www.indiatoday.in/india/story/tamil-nadu-unable-to-handle-stress-of-online-classes-student-dies-by-suicide-1718084-2020-09-03.

[7] "India's Online Fashion Market to Grow 3.5x from $4 Billion to $14 Billion by 2020, Marketing & Advertising News, ET Brand Equity." *ETBrandEquity.Com*, https://brandequity.economictimes.indiatimes.com/news/business-of-brands/indias-online-fashion-market-to-grow-3-5x-from-4-billion-to-14-billion-by-2020/63313245. Accessed February 18, 2021.

[8] Wertz, Jia. "3 Emerging E-Commerce Growth Trends To Leverage In 2020." *Forbes*, August 1, 2020, https://www.forbes.com/sites/jiawertz/2020/08/01/3-emerging-e-commerce-growth-trends-to-leverage-in-2020/?sh=27d00bd56fee.

[9] Sherman, Natalie. "Zoom Sees Sales Boom amid Pandemic - BBC News." *BBC News*, June 2, 2020, https://www.bbc.com/news/business-52884782.

[10] Patra, Ishan. "Google Meet Sees 30-Fold Growth since January - The Hindu." *The Hindu*, May 20 May 2020, https://www.thehindu.com/sci-tech/technology/internet/google-meet-sees-30-fold-growth-since-january/article31631115.ece.

[11] "Medscape: Medscape Access." *Latest Medical News, Clinical Trials, Guidelines - Today on Medscape*, https://www.medscape.com/slideshow/2020-medical-student-report-6013282#2. Accessed February February 21. 2021.

[12] McCarthy, Niall. "Chart: COVID-19's Staggering Impact On Global Education | Statista." *Statista Infographics*, https://www.statista.com/chart/21224/learners-impacted-by-national-school-closures/. Accessed February February 21. 2021.

[13] "Reliance-Backed AJIO Is Riding the Indian e-Commerce Wave — Poses Tough Competition to Myntra | Business Insider India." *Business Insider*, November November 2, 2020, https://www.businessinsider.in/business/ecommerce/news/reliance-backed-ajio-is-riding-on-the-indian-e-commerce-wave-poses-tough-competition-to-myntra/articleshow/78996579.cms.

[14] Kent, Dominic. "Microsoft Teams Statistics – Tom Talks." *Tom Talks*, December December 14, 2020, https://tomtalks.blog/2020/12/microsoft-teams-statistics/.

[15] "How Amazon Makes Money: E-Commerce, Advertising, and the Cloud." *Investopedia*, https://www.investopedia.com/how-amazon-makes-money-4587523. Accessed February February 21, 2021.

SECTION 3. RESPONSIBILITIES: WE ALL ARE TOGETHER

In: Impacts and Implications of COVID-19 ISBN: 978-1-53619-670-2
Editors: Anand Sharma et al.

Chapter 6

POLICIES FOR COVID-19 IN INDIA: FROM ONE DAY 'JANATA CURFEW' TO VACCINATION DRIVE

Vibha Ojha[1,*], Harshita Ojha[2], Ravi Sharma[3], Kinjal Sharma[4] and Anand Sharma[5]

[1]Government Engineering College, Ajmer, India
[2]IITTM, Gwalior, India
[3]School of Law, Symbiosis, Pune, India
[4]Institute of Law, Nirma University, Ahmedabad, India
[5]School of Engineering and Technology, MUST, Lakshmangarh, India

ABSTRACT

Coronavirus spread worldwide, influencing the worldwide economy, hitting administration and manufacturing sectors, and colossal effects on the workforce. There is a great emergency and calls for phenomenal measures. Its effect on weak people and families now lining neediness may enlarge imbalance gaps and even dig in destitution individuals. With the new announcement of

---

* Corresponding Author's E-mail: vibha.ojha@gmail.com.

COVID-19 as a pandemic by the World Health Organization (WHO), numerous nations have summoned general health laws managing pandemics and scourges. The WHO has set out a global administrative structure to manage general health crises in the International Health Regulation, 2005.

The effect of COVID-19 in Asia-Pacific is colossal because of monetary exercises, socioeconomics, and urbanization. At this pivotal crossroads when pretty much all aspects of the globe are inundated by the deadly COVID-19 pandemic, the current Indian government has stepped forward under Prime Minister Narendra Modi's authority by giving clinical help to a portion of its worldwide accomplices.

The government has reacted to the developing circumstance regarding general health and fears of financial slowdown by advising defensive measures through various services and offices managing the pertinent areas. This chapter shows the public authority's strategy proportions are being actualized through notice of fundamental amendments in law and are being refreshed or changed as the circumstance develops.

Keywords: COVID-19, SARS-CoV-2, quarantine, vaccine, vaccination drive, government policies

INTRODUCTION

The Covid-19 is brought about by SARS-CoV-2 "*Severe Acute Respiratory Syndrome Coronavirus-2*" [1, 2]. The degree of the implications caused is muddled, yet it is evident that the world has ground to a halt [3-5]. In the wake of the WHO "*World Health Organization*" on March 11, 2020, proclaiming COVID-19 a pandemic, and the ascent in revealed COVID-19 cases inside India, the reaction of the Government of India to the general public health crisis has been prompt, with a few notices being issued by the Central govt. and State govt., commanding lockdown and coordinating the closure of all, aside from recognized essential services.

India summoned a frontier law, *Epidemic Diseases Act, 1897* to combat coronavirus; the vast majority understood that it is in the literature. The pandemic in the 2020s digital age doesn't require such provincial law but warrants another public solid health ordinance. Is

India's administrative and legislative structure outfitted to manage such circumstances? The ordinance focuses on the combination of laws identifying with the guideline and counteraction of diseases. It is critically advanced for the control of the coronavirus spread.

The guideline guided all administration and private medical organizations to separate corners and screening forms for distinguishing cases. What's more, clinical officials and the administration must work as a team with state coordinated surveillance program workplaces. The guideline also worried about information/data hygiene — no individual/institute/association will utilize any print/digitally or web-based social networking to spread any data concerning COVID-19 without learning the official's realities and earlier clearance.

To control the spread of coronavirus in India, the Prime Minister declared nationwide lockdown for 21 days from March 25 to April 1o after one day of 'Janata Curfew' on March 22, 2020. On April 14, 2020 various states appealed to extend the lockdown to effectively tackle the pandemic. After this appeal by the states, the lockdown was extended nationwide until May 3, 2020, with some conditional relaxation after April 20 for the areas where the spread was in control. India's citizens and the government continue to fight the rising cases of Covid-19 with a nationwide lockdown [6].

The Ministry of Home Affairs (MHA), on May 1, 2020, posted an exhaustive review of the circumstances and gave an Order under the Disaster Management Act, 2005, to further extend the lockdown for a time of about fourteen days past May 4, 2020, until May 17. And three zones were across the country — Green Zone, Red Zone, and Orange Zone, with Red being the most dangerous and infected zone and to have the most impenetrable guidelines. Unwinding will be permitted in like manner.

At the national level, The *National Disaster Management Guidelines, 2008* attempted to overcome any health guidelines issues by keeping the *Ministry of Health and Family Welfare* as the nodal service.

The *National Health Bill, 2009* was a milestone in the health segment. Be that as it may, tragically, it didn't get changed over into an act. This Bill was focused on assurance and satisfaction of rights comparable to health, well-being, value equity, and justice. This proposed health services for all and the government's proactive job in accomplishing that objective.

MEASURES NOTIFIED BY INDIAN GOVERNMENT

On March 11, 2020, the *Indian government* gave a request to assign its capacity to *the Secretary* of *Ministry of Health and Family Welfare, Government of India,* to upgrade the readiness and control of COVID-19 and other auxiliary associated matters [7].

On the headings of Prime Minister Mr. Narendra Modi, the Group of Ministers (GOM) were "established to audit, screen and assess the readiness and measures taken to the executives" of novel coronavirus ailment (COVID-19) in the nation. The Ministry of Health and Family Welfare (MoHFW) planned the local Government's endeavors "to relieve the effect of the flare-up in India." On March 11, 2020, the GOM concluded that the MoHFW ought to exhort all state and association regions to summon segment 2 of the *Epidemic Disease Act, 1897*, with the goal that all warnings being given by the MoHFW, the states, and union territories, are enforceable.

The critical measures notified by the government can be categorized as:

- Modifying foreign investment approach to check astute takeovers and acquisitions of Indian organizations and mandating nationwide lockdown but notifying measures to enable movement of essential goods and services;
- Recognizing disruptions due to COVID-19 in performance of contractual obligations and providing for relief by permitting invocation of force majeure clauses or through exemption from penalties;
- Permitting lending institutions to grant a moratorium of three months on term loans and working capital facility-related reliefs.
- Extending the time for compliance by companies (for example, under Companies Act, 2013, tax laws and under labor laws);

- Advising public and private sector establishments to not terminate employees or deduct salaries for all employees, including casual and contract workers;
- Protecting micro, small and medium enterprises by increasing the default threshold for initiating corporate insolvency under the Insolvency and Bankruptcy Code to Rs. 1,00,00,000/- (Rupees One Crore);

Not at all like the Epidemic Disease Act has this law “accommodated a thorough authoritative set up for disaster readiness." On March 14, the union government announced COVID-19 as an informed calamity, and help is accessible under the State Disaster Response Fund (SDRF), which was built up likewise under the Disaster Management Act.

Quarantine Law Enforcement

In general healthcare practice, "quarantine" alludes to people's detachment (or networks) presented to an irresistible ailment. "Isolation," conversely, applies to the separation of people who are known to be contaminated. In quarantine, the irresistibly ill individuals are put in isolation for a fixed period to curd the infection's further spread. Coronavirus is exceptionally infectious; that’s why the people coming from the corona infected countries and the people interacting with the incoming travelers are being held under perception to determine their clinical status.

Verifiably, *India* has embraced the customary law solutions for quarantine enforcement, compelling amid pandemics. India also has exposed individuals to legally quarantine enforceable. It is in this setting relief and controls of the outburst of COVID-19 in India are along these lines of central significance, not exclusively to India yet to the world. The Ministry of Health and Family Welfare drafted a Public Health bill in 2017 for Control, Prevention, Epidemics Management, Bio-psychological terrorism, and Disasters to engage nearby government bodies for making a quick move during crisis circumstances.

The IPC "*Indian Penal Code*" manages offenses influencing the public health safety accommodation, respectability, and ethics that can be part into two significant parts:

i. Managing the quarantine rule,
ii. Managing the open aggravation.

The Epidemic Diseases Act additionally enhances the IPC law. Section 271 provides punishment of either depiction for a term that may stretch out to a half year, or with fine, or both for disobedience to any quarantine rule. Section 269 depicts "whosoever illegally or imprecisely does any manifestation which is, and which he knows or has a motivation to accept to be, prone to spread the contamination of any sickness hazardous to life, will be punished with the detainment of either depiction as long as a half year or fine or with both fine and detainment" [8].

The importance of the precedent-based law cure in this setting is an unusual request in recent speech from the viewpoint of access to medicines, health care services, and helpful impression of clinical conveyance. The arrangement of an open disturbance under Section 268 of the IPC visualizes that an individual is guilty of an open irritation when he does a demonstration that causes any primary injury, impediment, risk, or inconvenience to general society.

PM CARES FUND

Considering the COVID-19 pandemic situation in India, "the Prime Minister's Citizen Assistance and Relief in Emergency Situations Fund (PM CARES Fund)" was made on March 28, 2020. The asset will be utilized to battle, control, and aid projects against the COVID-19 outburst and comparative pandemic-like circumstances. The Prime Minister is the chairman of the trust. Trustees incorporate the Defense, Finance, and Home Ministers [9].

The asset will likewise empower micro-donations. It will fall under Corporate Social Responsibility (CSR) and will be charged absolved. The Prime Minister also stated that the PMO had gotten numerous solicitations to help in the battle against COVID-19. Likewise, the asset was set up and utilized for fiasco the board and exploration [10]. The Ministry of Corporate Affairs, Government of India, declared that donations made to this fund would fall under the organization's CSR commitment, with extra CSR being counterbalanced in resulting years.

Moreover, the Revenue Department of the Ministry of Finance mentioned its workers to obligatorily give a solitary day's salary to the asset consistently till March 2021. The workers were mentioned to give a composed application if they were not able to contribute.

AAROGYA SETU APP

Aarogya Setu App, the public authority's Covid-19 contact tracing application, could end up being the mother of all applications identified with the infection episode. The purpose of the Aarogya Setu App is to enlarge the Government of India's activities, especially the Department of Health, making people aware of the dangers around them, giving warnings, and giving information about best practices to control COVID-19.

As a feature of its endeavors to battle the lethal infection, the government dispatched the application Aarogya Setu, which means Health Bridge, a Bluetooth and GPS-based framework created by the country's National Informatics Center [11]. The application cautions clients who may have interacted with individuals later discovered to be positive for COVID-19 or considered to be in great danger. It must be utilized in state-claimed and private workplaces, and businesses should guarantee it is.

The application is accessible on Google Play Store. The application goes about as a one-stop answer for spreading mindfulness about COVID-19, assisting self with diagnosing clients, giving most recent updates, and even storing and showing e-pass. Notwithstanding, the most significant capacity is to follow contacts and make a dependable organization for the public authority to recognize potential COVID-19 casualties.

SUPREME COURT OF INDIA ANNOUNCEMENT – VIRTUAL HEARING

The judicial system is also heavily affected due to the shutdown of all the courts, from lower courts to the Supreme Court. The pandemic forced everything, businesses, jobs, education, etc., to change their manner from traditional to digital or virtual. After some time of lockdown, everything got again started but on online platforms virtually.

The SC *"Supreme Court of India"* has declared that from March 16, 2020, the Supreme Court will be dealing only with urgent and critical matters. The Supreme Court has also coordinated that lone the lawyers should follow up on the issue either for contentions or making oral contentions or help, alongside one prosecutor, will only be allowed in the court. The Supreme Court has likewise maintained all authority to require body temperature screening at all contestants and deny sections to people found to have body heat level.

In the first week of April 2020, seeing the delay in providing justice, the Apex Court of India also issued an order under Article 142 of the Constitution of India to hold the hearings of Courts virtually.

Article 142 provides power to the Supreme Court of India to issue any decree or order in any matter in which it thinks fir to provide justice.

Virtual hearing can be said as a legal hearing in a digital courtroom. It is done on an online platform on which the advocates and qualified judges discuss the matter online without appearing in the physical courtroom. It is the concept of adjudication of cases online to eliminate litigants' or lawyers' physical presence.

Only those matters that are urgent were taken to be discussed online, but now all the matters are being taken in virtual hearing. And now, not only the Supreme Court, almost all the High Courts are functioning online. A lot of problems are also there in this online system. Judges, advocates, parties and witnesses, etc., all face many difficulties in virtual hearing. But this pandemic left no other option in front of Courts to function.

This digitization or virtual hearing concept's biggest problem is the Information Technology (IT) infrastructure of courts in India. The internet connectivity in our country is not that good. And for video conferencing, only internet connection is not enough, speed of the Internet must also be good so that it can be done efficiently, and these facilities are not available in various courts and with many advocates. This is why the trial courts or the lower courts are not functioning online because the lower courts do not have the digital-friendly infrastructure. Some of the trial courts, where the situation is not as bad as they were during the pandemic, are started to open physically, and where the situation is not good, these courts are still not functioning.

The other problems with this are the connectivity issues, unfriendly nature of the judges and many advocates with this new system, cyber-security, etc. It has been challenging for judges and many advocates to conduct hearing online because of connectivity issues. If the internet connection is not very good or any other hindrance comes while the hearing is going on, it causes trouble in hearing, such as delay in hearing or lag in video and audio while arguments or while recording witnesses of witnesses. And due to this, the lack of confidence of the advocates while pleading is a significant drawback from the advocate's point of view.

Unfriendliness with this new system also causes a lot of trouble during the hearing as the judges and many lawyers are not very tech-savvy or digital-friendly. Many times, it has been seen that the judges lost their patience during the hearing while figuring this system out, and lawyers also forgot to turn the mic or video on or off at a particular time, causing a disturbance and making the situation awkward during the hearing.

Cyber-security is one of the significant issues faced in almost every sector during this digitization era [12]. This e-court and virtual hearing is a huge issue that must be dealt with very strictly. Almost all the essential documents are submitted or shown online in these virtual hearings, so the risk of getting these documents leaked is very high, and also the risk of getting these hearings hacked by a third party is also there.

The present battle against the COVID-19 pandemic may require measures that limit our human rights and significant freedoms, including the privilege to information insurance. In this regard, review that information security can in no way be a deterrent to sparing lives and that the material standards consistently consider an adjusting of the interests in question.

The pandemic renders people and society very vulnerable in all regards, while all depend like never on PC frameworks, cell phones, and the Internet. Malicious characters are exploiting these vulnerabilities furthering their potential benefit.

Criminal justice specialists are occupied with full participation to investigate, distinguish, detect, examine, property, and prosecute the related offenses and bring to justice those that misuse the COVID-19 pandemic for criminal purposes.

SUPPLY CHAIN MANAGEMENT

Specified the Supply chain disturbance brought about by the pandemic, all things considered, exhibitions under numerous agreements will be deferred, interrupted, interfered with, or even dropped [13]. Counterparties (particularly providers) to such agreements may look to postpone or potentially keep away from execution (or non-performing liability) of their contractual duties0and additionally end contracts, whichever because COVID-19 has genuinely kept them from playing out their authoritative commitments or because they are trying to blame it for removing themselves from a negative arrangement [14].

Force majeure related language utilized in many agreements shifts generally, and, in this manner, it is critical to review these provisions cautiously. A Force majeure condition can't be inferred under *Indian law*. This must be explicitly accommodated under the agreement, and insurance managed will rely upon the article's language [15].

Most agreements give that to an occasion to qualify as force majeure, which must be unforeseeable or not sensibly predictable at the agreement's execution time.

CRISIS COMMUNICATION STRATEGY

The viability of any crisis communication strategy, particularly during general well-being or public health disasters, relies similarly upon the exactness of data spread and its inclusivity. As the term 'communication' is expressive, the message's interpretation and receptivity vary for different groups.

The spread of the pandemic COVID-19 has affected the whole world; it affected not only public health systems but also crisis communications. The key in dealing with such a pandemic is clear, end-to-end crisis communication with diverse target groups through the primary medium of information consumption, i.e., social media.

With the rapid growth of digital communication channels, a national management framework was charted out by amending and expanding these legislations.

The World Health Organization (WHO) has praised the endeavors made by the Indian government in managing the coronavirus emergency.

The COVID-19 emergency is delivering exceptional difficulties for the varying audiovisual sector.

Because of this, legislatures, governments, and industry bodies are getting measures to help the different enterprises and their experts through this pandemic.

National Informatics Centre (NIC) Video Conferencing Services bolstered the meeting of Hon'ble Minister for Law & Justice, with Solicitor General, Attorney General, and all the Law Officers of Government of India (GoI). He accentuated to accept lockdown as an open the door to make advanced digital systems in justice delivery increasingly powerful.

Human Resource Management Policy

This, COVID-19, influences numerous people, regularly the least generously compensated and those self-employed or doing job in casual situations in the concert economy or low maintenance work with zero-hours contracts. The government has affirmed financial measures to defend jobs, ensure wages and bolster the self-employed [16].

Employees assume a massive role in the corporate segment. Indian laws exist to ensure employees and workers are dealt with well in workplaces and help secure their privileges. Employers are commonly committed to guaranteeing a sheltered and healthy workplace for their working professionals and must achieve 'everything sensibly conceivable' to guarantee avoidance of COVID-19 outbreak in the working environment [17]. An employer may forestall his employee who is experiencing COVID-19 type transmittable maladies from entering the working environment to secure different employees.

It confirms not to fire any employee because he/she is infected or is likely to be infected by a coronavirus.

There is the probability that State Governments may force further limitations on movement inside the state or city, if vital. In certain states, the employees of IT companies are directed to work from home.

Consequently, if the idea of work doesn't expect employees to be truly present, the prescribed strategy guarantees that every employee works from home, regardless of whether this isn't according to the typical policy of the establishment.

Information relating to the history of the person or medical status will establish delicate individual information, and assent ought to be taken by employees for disclosure as allowed under the applicable law and privacy policy. There is adequate language offered terms of employment (or worker handbooks) around direct well-being checks or moves being made to guarantee the representative's safety and security. In such a circumstance, it might be depended on to surmise assent. Extra assents might be gotten varying.

TRAVEL, TRANSPORTATION, AND IMMIGRATION POLICY

The Indian travel industry is crippled by the cascading effect of the coronavirus at a bewildering pace. The travel and tourism economy has been heavily affected by the coronavirus. The coronavirus outbreak also caused the cancellation of a lot of domestic and international flights.

Travel limitations, border shutdowns, and a decrease in flights have an immediate, extreme effect on worldwide travel in 2020. All significant visit administrators have declared an all-out suspension of activities. There has been a decrease in the number of homegrown explorers as individuals with business reasons or crisis necessities are just voyaging. Lockdowns and restricted interest networks to briefly close properties and forgo crossing out expenses for existing and new appointments at all their properties.

Hotels, eateries, vacation destinations, meeting and show settings, journey lines, aircraft, travel services, visit administrators, to give some examples, stopped to work or shortened their activity to a small portion of their ability. A vast number of individuals lost their positions, and a great many organizations will fail.

The Government of India has issued a few guidelines relating to travel limitations because of COVID-19 [18]. Notwithstanding visa limitations as of now set up, the people who traveled or visited Korea or France, or Italy and coming back to India will require an accurate report of tested negative for coronavirus from the affiliated labs' facilities approved by the health specialists of concerned nations. This was imposed from March 10, 2020, and is an impermanent measure until coronavirus cases die down. Any outside national who plans to venture out to India for any convincing explanation may contact the closest Indian Mission.

Every single approaching traveler, including Indian nationals, who are from or have visited China, the Republic of Korea, Iran, Spain, France, Italy, and Germany or any other highly infected nation from coronavirus after February 15, 2020, will be quarantined for a base time of fourteen days. This became effective on March 13, 2020, at the port of takeoff. Approaching explorers are encouraged to maintain a strategic distance from trivial travel and are educated to be isolated for at least fourteen days on their appearance in India.

Indian nationals are emphatically encouraged to desist heading out to China, the Republic of Korea, Italy, Iran, Spain, Germany, and France.

VACCINATION DRIVE

Refined hypotheses and great strategies are regularly baffled in their experience with realities and execution measures in the field. As of late uncovered, India's COVID-19 vaccine policy should take care not to travel that way and consider fundamental ground factors that could deliver nothing all around laid plans. With a complete fix not yet accessible for COVID-19, vaccines present the world with the best technique to back the infection off in its tracks alongside a proportion of vested group resistance, as SARS-CoV-2 frenzies on. While it may not be the enchantment wand, immunizing individuals will be the solitary known method of easing back the walk of the infection, and each nation, down to every district, should plan for this gigantic exercise. As the UK, what's more, the US started vaccinating their kin, India has declared its arrangement and proposed line-up for COVID-19 vaccination, not long after the Union Health Minister rejected that the public authority had at any point focused on COVID-19 vaccination for all in the country. According to the public authority's system, the vaccination is to be offered first to medical care workers and individuals beyond 50 years old, those more than 60 given priority, considering the circumstance. This will add up to around 30 crore individuals. The list of voters for the Lok Sabha and Assembly election polls has been set as the checking report for the interaction. Another computerized platform, Co-WIN, will be utilized for COVID-19 vaccination conveyance, and about 1.54 lakh Auxiliary Nurse Midwives chipping away at Universal Immunization Programmes will be roped in as vaccinators, with all the more such field staff to be activated in a joint effort with the States. Cold chain frameworks are to be reinforced the nation over to convey numerous dosages.

As governments meat up the vaccination drive, they need to clear the haze on vaccine safety and adequacy among individuals. With spending days, it won't be an excessive amount to anticipate from the public authority a detailed arrangement for vaccinating youngsters and a separate of errands down to the most reduced administration rung, as provinces in the US have been doing. Except if the last is done, an appropriate gauge of the genuine difficulties of overseeing antibodies in the field won't be accessible, and being ill-equipped is an assurance to coming fixed. Vaccine reluctance is a reality, and the best way to counter that will be transparent about unfriendly impacts and post-vaccination sequelae, assuming any, and disclose accessible, pertinent data in the domain. Before, in certain States, vaccination programs have endured incidentally because of deception about antagonistic occasions following shots. What's more, long-haul follow-up of all who get the immunization is significant for this situation. In that lies the affirmation that each one in the worldwide line list is sitting tight for.

Likewise, Supportive Supervision is dynamic help by the vaccine program administrators during the planning stage and implementation period of COVID-19 vaccine turn out at each level. The goal of supportive supervision is certainty and limit the working of colleagues to guarantee that Standard Operating Procedures being followed. State and different districts will send directors exceptionally for high danger/helpless performing locale and blocks. For a three to five vaccination group, a supervisor will be sent for close oversight at the session site. A portion of groups to supervisor will rely on separating of vaccination session and travel time.

Supervisors working in sloping and hard to arrive at regions may have more minor groups, while those working in blocked territories may have more groups. Group Supervisors will be furnished with normalized agenda and guide hands-on revisions/training to vaccination colleagues. A group-level supervisor's agenda is an essential tool for ongoing management.

Conclusion

The COVID-19 pandemic in *India* is moderately new contrasted with different nations. Appropriate observation and precise detailing of the attributes of contaminated people must happen. When an enormous extent of the world is in lockdown, the nations' economies are also affected very much. Without a vaccine promptly accessible to confine the outspread, Governments and global associations must concoct an emergency course of action.

The government of India is trying to find ways to fight this worldwide pandemic. The main element in preventing the outspread of the infection in local areas is by avoiding potential risk, considering the Ministry of Health and Family Welfare's warnings, and visiting the nearest medical center to test the infection in case you have coronavirus related manifestations.

The government has set up the best systems for numerous pinnacles. Indeed, even with the quick quarantine orders, revelation of national disaster, & the country lockdown, there are a viable legal mechanisms and alternate course of action to address the difficulties presented by COVID-19 and now the vaccination policies.

While the full effect of the Coronavirus flare-up on organizations isn't apparent right now, the episode will probably grow in the coming time, and it is getting basic continuously. This chapter has examined numerous issues featured in legitimate ramifications and Government strategies corresponding to the COVID-19 effect.

References

[1] World Health Organization (2020). *Report of the WHO-China Joint Mission on Coronavirus Disease 2019 (COVID-19).* Available online at https://www.who.int/docs/default-source/coronaviruse/who-china-joint-mission-on-covid-19-final-report.pdf.

[2] Madaan, V, A Roy, C Gupta, P Agrawal, A Sharma, C Bologa, R Prodan. (2021). XCOVNet: Chest X-ray Image Classification for COVID-19 Early Detection Using Convolutional Neural Networks. *New Generation Computing,* pp. 1-15, 2021. doi: 10.1007/s00354-021-00121-7.

[3] Agrawal, Akshat, Rajesh Arora, Ranjna Arora, Prateek Agrawal. (2021). Applications of Artificial Intelligence and Internet of Things for Detection and Future Directions to Fight against COVID-19. In edited book on *Emerging Technologies for Battling Covid-19,* pp. 107-119, Springer.

[4] Agrawal, Prateek, Vishu Madaan, Aditya Roy, Rajani Kumari & Harshal Deore. (2021). FOCOMO: Forecasting and monitoring the worldwide spread of COVID-19 using machine learning methods, *Journal of Interdisciplinary Mathematics*, pp. 1-25. DOI: 10.1080/09720502.2021.1885812.

[5] Huang C, Wang Y, Li X, et al. Clinical features of patients infected with 2019 novel coronavirus in Wuhan, China. *Lancet.* 2020;395(10223):497e506.

[6] Jin YH, Cai L, Cheng ZS, et al. A rapid advice guideline for the diagnosis and treatment of 2019 novel coronavirus (2019-nCoV) infected pneumonia (standard version). *Mil Med Res.* 2020;7(1):4.

[7] Campbell D, Bannock. *'Unlike Anything Seen in Peacetime': NHS Prepares for Surge in Covid-19 Cases*; 2020. https://www.theguardian.com/world/2020/mar/13/unlike-anything-seen-in-peacetime-nhs-prepares-for-surge-in-covid-19-coronavirus-cases.

[8] Tarique Faiyaz, *COVID-19 and the Current Challenges of Quarantine Law Enforcement in India, JURIST – Student Commentary*, April 14, 2020, https://www.jurist.org/commentary/2020/04/tarique-faiyaz-covid-19-quarantine-india/.

[9] "PM Narendra Modi announces PM-CARES fund to fight coronavirus outbreak." *Business Standard India. PTI. March 29 2020*. Retrieved March 29 2020.

[10] "PM CARES Fund: All You Need to Know." *DATAQUEST. March 30 2020*. Retrieved July 18 2020.

[11] nic-delhi/AarogyaSetu_Android, nic-delhi, May 27 2020, retrieved 21July 2020.

[12] https://www.marketsandmarkets.com/Market-Reports/covid-19-impact-on-cybersecurity-market-128702677.html.

[13] McKibbin, W. and R. Fernando (2020) *The Global Macroeconomic Impacts of COVID-19: Seven Scenarios*. https://www.brookings.edu/research/the-global-macroeconomic-impacts-of-covid-19-seven-scenarios/.

[14] Baldwin, R. and BW. Di Mauro 2020. Economics in the Time of Covid-19. *CEPR*. https://voxeu.org/content/economics-time-covid-19.

[15] https://doe.gov.in/sites/default/files/Force%20Majeure%20Clause%20-FMC.pdf.

[16] Lee, A. and J. Cho 2016. *The impact of epidemics on labor market: identifying victims of the Middle East Respiratory*.

[17] ILO (2018) *Care work and care jobs for the future of decent work*. ILO, Geneva.

[18] Chinazzi M, Davis JT, Ajelli M, et al. The effect of travel restrictions on the spread of the 2019 novel coronavirus (COVID-19) outbreak. *Science*. 2020. https://doi.org/10.1126/science.aba9757.

In: Impacts and Implications of COVID-19 ISBN: 978-1-53619-670-2
Editors: Anand Sharma et al.

Chapter 7

COMPARATIVE ANALYSIS OF COVID-19 VACCINE CANDIDATES

Amit Kumar Verma[1,*],
Divyank Awasthi[2] and Preeti Mishra[3]
[1]Department of Pharmacy, MJP Rohilkhand University, Bareilly U.P., India
[2]Varun Arjun Medical & Pharmacy College, Bareilly U.P., India
[3]Raja Balwant Singh Engineering Technical Campus Bichpuri Agra, U.P., India

ABSTRACT

The mysterious virus SARS-CoV-2 originated in Wuhan, China, resulting in the coronavirus disease 2019 (COVID-19) turn out into a pandemic. On January 11, 2020, the most awaited genome sequence of the SAR COV-2 was released. After that, SARS-CoV-2 genome sequences were released by China CDC; this created the new path for the development of the diagnostic kit, therapeutic agents, and most important, vaccine. Till January 26, 2021, 63 vaccine candidates are in clinical development, and 174 candidates

* Corresponding Author's E-mail: professoramitmjpuniversity@gmail.com.

are in preclinical development. Twenty vaccine candidates are using the protein subunit platform, which is 32% of the total vaccine platform used. The candidates of the vaccine are using a viral vector (non-replicating), DNA, Inactivated virus, RNA, viral vector (replicating), etc. In terms of dosage and schedule, 38 vaccine candidates are using two doses while 53 vaccine candidates are following the injectable route of administration.

Keywords: SARS-CoV-2, COVID-19, patient, vaccines

INTRODUCTION

On January 11, 2020, the most awaited genome sequence of the SAR COV-2 was released. After that, SARS-CoV-2 genome sequences were released by China CDC; this created the new path for the development of the diagnostic kit, therapeutic agents, and most important, vaccine. The biological entity which can generate an immune response to a particular antigen or foreign substance usually derived from any pathogen.

Edward Jenner was remembered to develop or introduce the first vaccine in 1796, incorporating cowpox to inoculate against disease caused by cowpox. The concept worked well; thus, till the time they are helpful in removing or eradicating the various infectious disease from particular area Vaccine candidates have multiple target antigens such four structural proteins of coronaviruses such S protein, envelope (E) protein, membrane (M) protein, and nucleocapsid (N) protein) [1]. The immune response is mediated mainly by S type protein, this protein viz angiotensin-converting enzyme 2 (ACE-2) is required for host cell entry [2-7]."The binding of the S protein to the ACE-2 receptor triggers complex conformational changes, driving the S protein from a prefusion conformation to a post-fusion conformation. The decoration of the post-fusion conformation with N-linked glycans was suggested as a potential strategy for the virus to evade the host immune response" [8]. This chapter presents the comparative analysis of several COVID-19 vaccines on the basis of their status in trial phases, route of administration, dosage, efficacy, and safety.

DESIGNING OF COVID-19 VACCINES

In the initial stage of virus spread, many pieces of research were done to predict the impact [9, 10]. Later, researchers put their efforts into early diagnosis of the infection [11], and in parallel to that, the researchers also started finding solutions to develop the vaccines to counter the virus. There are many types of vaccines that are under trial or development to address the emergency situation of COVID-19. The types may include vaccines based on inactivation, RNA/DNA vaccines, vector-based vaccines, a vaccine based on live attenuation, vaccines having recombinant subunits as well as those based on viral particles too.

Viruses turn to non-infectious or inactivated using physical or chemical techniques and are presented through numerous viral proteins for immune recognition, show stability and easy production in enormous quantities [12]. Traditionally inactivated viruses after purification has been traditionally used for vaccine development and are equally effective in combating the disease; for example, influenza virus, vaccines based on live attenuation have shown promising results in curing infections, for example, smallpox and poliomyelitis [13].

DNA/RNA Vaccine or Nucleic Acid Vaccines

Vaccines having either DNA or RNA, such as mRNA vaccines and DNA vaccines, are commonly used vaccine format. These are incorporated into human cells, where they will then be transcribed into viral proteins. Out of all coronavirus proteins, the most common aspirant is S-type protein. Due to the advantages of increased potency, cheapness, rapid production of mRNA, vaccines are preferred over conventional vaccines [14, 15]. In terms of therapeutic efficacy, DNA vaccines also have great higher potential due to their capacity to increase T-cell induction & antibody production, the excellent biocompatibility of plasmid deoxyribonucleic acid, cheap manufacturing, and they prolong shelf life [16]. Low immunogenicity is actually the disadvantage of this DNA-based vaccine, and the problem of crossing the nuclear membrane is a matter of concern.

Vector Vaccines

Carrier virus help in the construction of vector-based vaccines. Carrier viruses such as adeno or pox virus are modified for the incorporation of a particular gene from the virus; the S gene may be the part obtained for coronaviruses. "The key advantage of vector vaccines is that the immunogen is expressed in the context of a heterologous viral infection, which induces the innate immune responses required for the adaptive immune responses" [17].

Subunit Vaccines and Virus-Like Particles Vaccines

In this type of vaccine, viral-based proteins are administered into the host tissue to determine the potentiality of the protection in humans from viral infection. The antigenic complexity of the virus, in this case, is not fully explored as there is the only incorporation of few parts, the possibility of unwanted lethal immune reaction cannot be ignored [18].

Neutralizing Antibodies Types

Antibodies of neutralizing type proved to display a crucial role in inhibiting the infection of viral nature [19]. Monoclonal antibodies (mAbs) are the top choice in this format due to various advantages; however other formats also include such as antibodies having single-domain, single-chain variable fragments (scFvs), and functional antigen-binding fragments (Fabs).

The isolation of monoclonal antibodies can be done from recovered patients having virus infection previously or from immunized transgenic animal models that are immunized, Neutralizing antibodies, particularly those targeting the RBD of SARS-CoV-2, may serve as a promising targeted therapeutic way to viral infection [20, 21].

Vaccine Production and Their Clinical Trial

An unexpected outbreak of COVID-19 and searching for vaccine solutions provokes many countries such as China, Russia to start to administer the vaccine before the completion of the phase three trial; however, there is a possibility of severe side effects in the long term. A total of one hundred and seventy-four vaccines in preclinical development and sixty-three vaccines in clinical development are involved. The candidates for the clinical trial are based on various platforms involving protein subunit, viral vector (replicating) inactivated virus, DNA, RNA virus vector-non replicating, virus-like particle, virus-like particle, live attenuated virus, viral vector replicating & antigen-presenting cell, and viral vector non-replicating & antigen-presenting cell. Various vaccines have been produced by various developers [22].

Sinovac Research and Development Co. Ltd.

The random trial is performed to determine the efficiency and safety of inactivated virus platform in the phase-III trial of this intravenous vaccine; two-dose in intramuscular mode with an interval of fourteen days is involved. The study of efficacy is based on the detection of symptoms of SARS-CoV-2 infection after the first and second doses of the vaccine. For safety measurement, different age groups like adults (involving 18 to 59 years) and elders (more than 50 years) are involved. The observation time is up to twelve months.

Sinopharm, China National Biotec Group Co. & Wuhan Institute of Biological Products

After the random placebo-based trials, this inactivated virus platform-based inactivated SARS – CoV-2 vaccine (Vero cell) vaccine in under Phase-III trial for both efficacies as well safety. In the (0 to 21) days duplicate dose where the route of administration is intramuscular in phase-I and phase-2 trial, a low rate of adverse reaction is observed.

Sinopharm, China National Biotech Group Co. & Beijing Institute of Biological Products

It is also an inactivated SARS-CoV-2 vaccine (Vero cell) and comes in inactivated virus platform. Two intramuscular doses with an interval of twenty-one days are required. The phase-III trial will be based on a randomized, double-blind study for immunogenicity and safety.

Astra Zeneca & University of Oxford

The viral vector (non-replicating) Ch Ad Ox – 1-S (AZD 1222) Covishield), a vaccine with two doses at 28 days intervals by the intramuscular route of administration, is under phase 3 trial. Encouraging results are obtained from phase one and phase two trials.

CanSino Biological Inc./Beijing Institute of Biotechnology

The vaccine developed by this company is a viral vector (Non replicating) type recombinant novel coronavirus vaccine (Adenovirus type 5 vector); only one dose is suggested by an intramuscular method. Phase III trial is under study for safety and immunogenicity.

Gamaleya Research Institute Health Ministry and the Russian Federation

The viral vector (non-replicating) Gam. COVID-Vac adeno-based (r Ad 26-S + r Ad-5-S) vaccine. It is used intramuscularly in two doses at the interval of 21 days. It is also in phase 3 trial after getting the positive results for efficacy and immunity lest. ELISA-based measurements by antibody level determination have been used for phase 1 and phase 2 trials. The phase 3 trial will be done.

Janssen Pharmaceutical

It is a vaccine with a viral vector of non-replicating type Ad 26.CoV2.5 with 1-2 days, one at zeroth day and another after fifty-sixth days intramuscularly. This is also in the phase III trial.

Novavax

Novavax has produced an intramuscularly injectable protein submit, SARS-CoV-2rS/Matrix M1- Adjuvant (Full-length recombinant SARS CoV-2 glycoprotein nanoparticle vaccine adjuvant with matrix M) vaccine. Two doses of vaccine at the interval of 21 days are requested. This is also in the phase III trial.

Moderna National Institution of Allergy and Infected Diseases (NIAID)

The vaccine is of RNA vaccine platform and based on m-RNA-1273 and requires two intramuscular doses with a difference of 28 days. This is also under study for Phase-III trial regarding effectiveness, safety, and reactogenicity.

Pfizer/Bio-NTech & Fosun Pharma

The vaccine requires two doses of intramuscular injection at 0 days and after 21 days. 97 is an RNA-based vaccine and under a third phase trial study based on BNT 162 (3 LNP-m RNA).

Anhul Zhifei Longcom Biopharmaceutical and Institute of Microbiology, Chinese Academy of Sciences

The vaccine is a protein subunit based on recombinant: SARS-CoV-21 vaccine (CHO cell). It requires two to three doses with 28 days intervals of 0, 28, and 56 days intramuscular injection. This is also in phase III trial for its safety and efficacy determination.

Cure Vac AG

This company produced a CVn CoV vaccine based on RNA and required intramuscular two doses with a difference of 28 days. The randomized placebo-controlled trial for phase III has been started.

Institute of Medical Biology and Chinese Science

The SARS-CoV-2 vaccine (Vero cells) vaccine is based on the inactivated virus and requires two intramuscular doses with 28 days interval. This is also under phase III trial.

Research Institute for Biological Safety Problem, Republic of Kazakhstan

Raz Covid-in[r] COVID-19 inactivated vaccine based on inactivated virus required two intramuscular injections at the interval of 21 days; it is in phase III trial.

Inovio Pharmaceuticals, International Vaccine Institute and AdVaccine (Suzhou) Biopharmaceutical Co. Ltd.

The IND-4800+ electroporation candidate-based on DNA-based vaccine requires two intradermal injections at the interval of 26 days and undergone in only phase II trial.

AnGes, Takare Bio & Ozaka Universkty

DNA-based, AGO 301-COVID 19 vaccine requires two intramuscular doses with 14 days intervals. Now, it is in phase 2/3 trial study for safety and effectiveness.

Zydus Cadila

It is an intradermal injectable, DNA-based, n CoV vaccine and requires three doses at 0, 28, and 56 days. It is in phase III trial.

Genexine Consortium

Gx-19 in a DNA base vaccine & requires two intramuscular doses with a difference of 28 days. This vaccine is in phase 1/2 trial.

Bharat Biotech International Ltd.

The whole virion inactivated SARS – CoV-2 vaccine (BBV 152) is an inactivated virus-based vaccine requiring two doses via intramuscular injection at 14 days intervals. This is in the phase III trial.

Keitucky Bioprocessing Inc.

It produced a KBP – COVID-19 (RBD-based) vaccine, which is based on protein submit. It requires two intramuscular doses with 21 days interval. It is under phase-1/2 trial.

Sanofi Pasteur & GSK

This Institute produced an intramuscular double dose vaccine candidate named SARS-CoV-2 vaccine formulation 1 with adjuvant 1 (S protein (baculovirus production) which is based on protein subunit. It is under phase-1/2 trial and requires two doses at 21 days intervals via intramuscular injection.

Areturus Therapeutics

ARC-021 is RNA based vaccine that requires intramuscular administration. Phase-III trials have been performed.

Serum Institute of India & Accelager Pty and Spy Biotech

The RBD SARS-CoV-2 HBs Ag VLP vaccine candidate is a virus-like particle type vaccine that requires two intramuscular injections at the interval of 28 days. This is under phase 1/2 trial.

Beijing Minhai Biotechnology Co.

This Institute produced inactivated, based on inactivating virus-based candidates, requires three intramuscular doses. It is under phase III trial.

Rei There, Leukocare and Univecells

The vaccine GRAd-COV-2 (Replication defective simian A dew virus (GRAd) encoding 5) is a viral vector non replicating type vaccine. It requires one intramuscular dose. It is under phase I trial.

Vaxart

The VXA-CoV2-1Ad5 adjuvanted oral vaccine platform is a viral vector non-replicating candidate. It is under phase I trial and requires oral administration of two doses with an interval of 28 days.

The University of Munich (Ludwig-Maximillian)

It also produced viral vector non-replicating type MVA-SARS-2-S vaccine. It also requires intramuscular two doses with an interval of 28 days. It is the phase-I trial study for safety as well as effectiveness.

Clover Bio Pharmaeuticals Inc./GSK. Dynavax

The vaccine candidate is SCB-2019+AS03 or CpG 1018 adjuvant plus alum adjuvant (Native like Trimeric subunit spike protein vaccine). It is a protein subunit-based vaccine. The vaccine is under phase 2/3 trial—this needs two intramuscular doses with a difference of 21 days.

Vaccine Pty Ltd.

The COVAX-19 recombinant spike protein + adjuvant vaccine is based on protein submit. It is under phase I trial; it need are intramuscular administration.

Medien Vaccine Biologics, Dynavax, and National Institute of Allergy and Infectious Diseases (NIAID)

MVC-COV1901 (S-2P protein + CPG 1018) is a protein subunit-based vaccine. It is under phase 2/3 trial. It requires intramuscular administration in two doses with an interval of 28 days.

Institute Finlay de Vaccines

The FINLAY-FRanti -SARS-CoV-2 vaccine (RBD + Adjuvant) vaccine candidate is a protein subunit-based candidate. It has completed phase two trial. The intramuscular two doses are required at an interval of 28 days.

Federal Budgetary Research Institution State Research center of Virology and Biotechnology "Vector"

A protein subunit-based candidate Epi VacCorona (Epi Vac Corona): Vaccine based on peptide antigens for the prevention of COVID-19 is produced by the developers. It has completed the phase I/II trial. It needs two successive intramuscular injections with an interval of 21 days.

West China Hospital & Sichuan University

These Institutes in their combined effort, develop protein subunit based, RBD (baculovirus) production expressed in S.F. 9 cells) Recombinant SARS-CoV-2 vaccine (S.F. 9 cells) candidate with two doses intramuscular administration mode within 28 days. It has completed phase II trial for it is efficacy and safety and safety norms.

University Hospital Tuebingen

The protein subunit-based, IMPCo Vac-1 (SAR-CoV-2 HLA-DR peptides) vaccine with a single dose and subcutaneous administration mode was developed, and it has completed the phase-I trial.

COVAXX and United Biomedical Inc.

These agencies developed UB-612 (Multimode peptide based S1-RBD – protein based vaccine it is available in two intramuscular doses within 28 days. Phase II/III trials for the immunogenicity and safety measures have been done.

University of Hong Kong, Xiamen University & Beijing Wantai Biological Pharmacy

Del NSI – 2019-n CoV-RBD-OPT-1 (Intranasal flu-based-RBD) vaccine, which comes in viral vector (replicating) category, has been developed with single-dose intranasal administration mode and has completed the phase-II trial.

Imperial College London

Another RNA-based LNP-n CoVsaRNA vaccine with intramuscular, double dose pattern has completed phase I trial for it is effectiveness as well as safety.

Academy of Military Science (AMS), Walvax Biotechnology and Suzhou Abogen Biosciences

These agencies co-operatively develop the RNA-based candidate, SARS-CoV-2 m RNA vaccine (A.R. CoV). It has a two-dose pattern for administration – either 0 and 14 days interval or 0 and 28 days interval and intramuscular mode is selected for this vaccine. It has completed its phase I trial.

Medicago Inc.

The Institute developed a virus-like particle base vaccine, Corona Virus-Like particle COVID-19 (Co VLP). It is under the phase II/III trial. Intramuscular mode with two successive doses at 0 and 21 days is suggested for clinical use.

Shenzhen Geno – Immune Medical Institute

The Covid-19//a APC vaccine. The candidate, Covid-19/a APC vaccine, is synthesized by involving the modification using immune-modulatory genes and viral minigenes to the artificial antigen-presenting cells (APCs). It involves subcutaneous mode in three doses (0, 14, and 28 days) for administration. It has completed the phase I trial.

Shenzhen Geno-Immune Medical Institute

The same Institute also develop a viral vector (Non-replicating) and APC-based, LV-SMENP-DC vaccine in this candidate; the modified dendrite cells with lentivirus vectors expressing COVID-19 mini gene SMENP and immune-modulatory genes are used. CTLS is activated using the LV-DC presenting COVID-19 specific antigens. It requires only one dose, either subcutaneously or by intravenous mode, for clinical application. It has completed phase I/II trial study.

Adimmune Corporation

Admire SC-2f recombinant RBD +/- Aluminum): a vaccine is a protein subunit-based candidate. It has completed the phase-I trial.

Entos Pharmaceutical Inc.

DNA-based candidate, Covigenix VAX-001-DNA vaccines with proteo-lipid vehicle (PLV) formulation is developed. It needs two doses within 14 days of interval in 1 M mode. The vaccine has completed the phase I trial.

Providence Health and Services

The agency developed another DNA-based vaccine, CORVax-Spike (S) protection plasmid DNA vaccine. It is administered by intradermal mode in two successive doses within the interval of 14 days and has completed a phase-I trial for clinical use.

Chulalongkorn University

The University has developed ChulaCoV-19 m RNA vaccine. It is an RNA-based candidate and needs two intramuscular doses at 0 and 21 days has completed it is phase-I trial studies.

Symvivo Corporation

The corporation prepared a DNA-based vaccine bac TRL-Spike oral DNA vaccine. As the name implies, it requires oral administration in a single dose and has successfully passed it is a phase-I trial for effectiveness and safeness study.

Immunity Bio, Inc & Nantkwest Inc.

The coordinative efforts of their institution developed a viral vector (Non-replicating vaccine h Ad 5-S. Fusion +N-ETSD vaccine. It can be given subcutaneously or by oral mode, and It has passed phase-I trial study.

City of Hope Medical Center and National Center Institute, The COHO4S1 (MVA-SARS-2-S)

Modified vaccine Ankara (& MVA) platform + synthetic SARS-CoV-2 vaccine has been developed which come under the viral (Non-replication) vaccines. It needs one to two-dose at the interval of 28 days by intramuscular mode. It has completed the phase I/II trial.

Israel Institute for Biological Research

The rVSV-SARS-CoV-2-S vaccine in viral vector (replicating) vaccine and needs a single intramuscular injection mode. It has successfully completed the phase I/II trial.

Aivita Biomedical, Inc. National Institute of Health Research and Development Ministry of the Health Republic of Indonesia

The combined effects of these institutions prepared viral vector (replicating) and APC-based candidate, Dendrite cell vaccine AV-COVID-19. In which the vaccine has dendrite cells having antigens from SARS-CoV-2, with or without GM-CSF. It is an intramuscular single-dose vaccine and completed phase I/II trial.

Codagenix/Serum Institute of India

The Cov 1-VAC is a live attenuated virus type vaccine that requires a one/two-dose administration pattern within 28 days intervals. It can be given by in mode. It has completed the phase I trial.

Center for Genetic Engineering and Biotechnology (CIGB)

CIGB-669 (RBD + Agn HB) vaccine development by this Institute is a protein subunit-based vaccine. It involves three doses at 1, 14, and 28 days intervals or 0, 28, and 56 days intervals by intramuscular mode.

Centre for Genetic Engineering and Biotechnology (CIGB)

This institution also developed another protein submit-based vaccine, CIGB-66 (RBD + aluminum hydroxide). Three intramuscular doses at 0, 14, and 28 days or at 0, 28, and 56 days is required. Phase I/II trial has been completed.

Valneva, National Institute for Health Research United Kingdom

The vaccine VLA 2001 is an inactivated virus-based vaccine. Two doses of the vaccine are required at the difference of 21 days by intramuscular mode. Phase I/II trial has been completed.

Biological E Ltd.

BE CoV-2 vaccine is a protein subunit-based vaccine developed by this Institute. It can be administered intramuscularly on day 0 and day 28 in two doses. Phase I or II trial has been completed.

Cellid Co. Ltd.

The Institute has developed an AdCLD-CoV19 (adenovirus vector) vaccine based on the viral vector (replicating). It needs only a single intramuscular dose. Phase I/II trial has been completed.

Gene One Life Science, Inc.

The agency has prepared a DNA based, GLS-5310 vaccine doses can be given either at 0 and 56 days or 0 and 84 day in I.D. mode administration. Phase I/II trial has been completed.

Nanogen Pharmaceutical Biotechnology

A protein submit-based, recombinant SARS-CoV-2 spike protein, Aluminum adjuvanted vaccine, has been developed. It can be given by two successive doses at the interval of 21 days in intramuscular mode. Phase I/II trial has successfully completed.

Shionogi

The Institute developed a protein submit-based candidate, recombinant protein vaccine S-268019 (using Baculovirus expansion vector system). This vaccine can be given intramuscularly in two doses at the interval of 21 days. Phase I/II trial has been completed.

Altimmune, Inc.

The Institute has developed a viral vector (non replicating) vaccine which requires a single dose by intramuscular mode. The Ad COVID, Adenovirus-based platform, expresses the receptor-binding domain

(RBD) of the SARS-CoV-2 spike protein. Phase I trial has been completed.

University Medical Center Groningen and Akston Bio Sciences Inc.

The research of these centers has developed a protein subunit-based vaccine, SARS-CoV-2-RBD-Fc fusion protein. It can be given either subcutaneous or intramuscular mode. Phase I/II trial has been completed.

Erciyes University

The inactivated virus-based vaccine has been developed. The ERUCOV-VAC, Inactivated virus vaccine, can be administered intramuscularly in two doses in two doses at a difference of 21 days. The trial for phase I has been completed.

Vaccine and Infectious Disease Organization (VIDO) and Septic and the Vaccine Formulation Institute (VFI)

The vaccine has completed phase I/II trial. It can be administered for 28 days.

CONCLUSION

The results of the clinical trial for the number confirmed cares of the disease, the % of effectiveness or compared to the placebo for prevention from the virus the data related to the efficiency of a vaccine against the severe and non-severe cases. For hospitalization, the need for ICU and the number of death are also under study. The results are awaited. The randomized study, including different age groups, different health statuses, sexes, etc., is involved in checking the safety as well as immunogenic power of the vaccines.

References

[1] Verma, A. K. et al. *COVID-19: A Drill-Down Analysis* Aug 2020; page no 14; Insc Publishing House, Karnataka, India.

[2] Zhou, P. et al. A pneumonia outbreak associated with a new coronavirus of probable bat origin. *Nature* 579, 270–273 (2020).

[3] Ou, X. et al. Characterization of spike glycoprotein of SARS-CoV-2 on virus entry and its immune cross-reactivity with SARS-CoV. *Nat. Commun.* 11, 1620 (2020).

[4] Hoffmann, M. et al. SARS-CoV-2 cell entry depends on ACE2 and TMPRSS2 and is blocked by a clinically proven protease inhibitor. *Cell* 181, 271–280.e8 (2020). Its S1 & S2 two subunits, S1 having RBD causing binding to ACE 2 receptor and cell membrane fusion, respectively.

[5] Letko, M., Marzi, A. & Munster, V. Functional assessment of cell entry and receptor usage for SARS-CoV-2 and other lineage B betacoronaviruses. *Nat. Microbiol.* 5, 562–569 (2020).

[6] Wan, Y. et al. Receptor recognition by the novel coronavirus from Wuhan: an analysis based on decade-long structural studies of SARS coronavirus. *J. Virol.* 94, e00127–20 (2020).

[7] Cai, Y. et al. Distinct conformational states of SARS-CoV-2 spike protein. *Science* 369, 1586–1592 (2020).

[8] Bisht, H. et al. Severe acute respiratory syndrome coronavirus spike protein expressed by attenuated vaccinia virus protectively immunizes mice. *Proc. Natl Acad. Sci.* USA 101, 6641–6646 (2004).

[9] Agrawal, Akshat, Arora, Rajesh, Arora, Ranjna, Agrawal, Prateek (2021). Applications of Artificial Intelligence and Internet of Things for Detection and Future Directions to Fight Against COVID-19. In edited book on *Emerging Technologies for Battling Covid-19,* pp. 107-119, Springer.

[10] Agrawal, Prateek, Madaan, Vishu, Roy, Aditya, Kumari Rajani, & Deore, Harshal (2021). FOCOMO: Forecasting and monitoring the worldwide spread of COVID-19 using machine learning methods, *Journal of Interdisciplinary Mathematics*, pp. 1-25. DOI: 10.1080/09720502.2021.1885812.

[11] Madaan, V., Roy, A., Gupta, C., Agrawal, P., Sharma, A., Bologa, C., Prodan, R. (2021). XCOVNet: Chest X-ray Image Classification for COVID-19 Early Detection Using Convolutional Neural Networks. *New Generation Computing,* pp. 1-15, 2021. DOI: 10.1007/s00354-021-00121-7.

[12] Roper, R. L. & Rehm, K. E. SARS vaccines: where are we? *Expert Rev. Vaccines* 8, 887–898 (2009).

[13] Minor, P. D. Live attenuated vaccines: historical successes and current challenges. *Virology* 479-480, 379–392 (2015).

[14] Pardi, N., Hogan, M. J., Porter, F. W. & Weissman, D. mRNA vaccines—a new era in vaccinology. *Nat. Rev. Drug Disco.* 17, 261–279 (2018).

[15] Wang, F., Kream, R. M. & Stefano, G. B. An evidence based perspective on mRNASARS- CoV-2 vaccine development. *Med Sci. Monit.* 26, e924700 (2020).

[16] Hobernik, D. & Bros, M. DNA Vaccines-How far from clinical use? *Int. J. Mol. Sci.* 19, 3605 (2018).

[17] Afrough, B., Dowall, S. & Hewson, R. Emerging viruses and current strategies for vaccine intervention. *Clin. Exp. Immunol.* 196, 157–166 (2019).

[18] Enjuanes, L. et al. Molecular basis of coronavirus virulence and vaccine development. *Adv. Virus Res* 96, 245–286 (2016).

[19] Lv, H. et al. Cross-reactive Antibody Response between SARS-CoV-2 and SARSCoV Infections. *Cell Rep.* 31, 107725 (2020).

[20] Lurie, N., Saville, M., Hatchett, R. & Halton, J. Developing Covid-19 vaccines at pandemic speed. *N. Engl. J. Med.* 382, 1969–1973 (2020).

[21] Wec, A. Z. et al. Broad neutralization of SARS-related viruses by human monoclonal antibodies. *Science* 369, 731–736 (2020).

[22] Clinicaltrials.gov (U.S. National Library of Medicines); *SARS CoV Data base.*

In: Impacts and Implications of COVID-19 ISBN: 978-1-53619-670-2
Editors: Anand Sharma et al.

Chapter 8

IMPLICATIONS OF COVID-19 IN INDIA: A JOURNEY FROM PHYSICAL TO DIGITAL

Arushi Gupta[1] and Pooja Kansra[2,*]
[1]Panjab University, Chandigarh, India
[2]Mittal School of Business, Lovely Professional University, Punjab, India

ABSTRACT

Life has gone for a toss during the coronavirus pandemic. New paths have been discovered, and old paths have been refurbished. The virus has been spreading and claiming lives daily. Not only the humans but the economy too is bearing the brunt of the virus. Pre-pandemic time, the economy was already grappling to make a turnabout and make a new start but, the onset of the lockdown in March has only exacerbated the situation. Some sectors are affected badly and some less. The economy sees contraction, growth rates in negative, lakhs of people forked out unemployed, etc. However, being optimistic is what gets us going. The economy may revive sooner than expected. Some sectors may revive early and some later. This research paper deals with the aftermath

* Corresponding Author's E-mail: pooja.kansra@gmail.com.

strategies to help the economy recover, the new definition of "new normal," the growth drivers sectors of the economy etc. It also deals with the various sectors of the affected economy such as aviation, infrastructure, health, hospitality, impacts and revival strategies. Every sector needs to be dealt with differently. We need to learn to live with the virus till the proper vaccination arrives for mass immunization.

In India, the pandemic has asserted for the provision of appropriate health care services, resilient infrastructure, health, and education is the topmost priority of the public and the private entities, a transformative role to be played by the hospitality sector, the pharmaceuticals sector being the game-changer. With the economy moving to the new normal, the government needs to devise such strategies to take the economy to a much-improved state, restoring lost jobs, a much-needed fiscal stimulus, and the economy to be "aatma-nirbhar" (self-resilient). The economy may soon witness a V-shaped recovery. There is an urgent need to augment drug production and medical devices, which can be achieved through the production-linked incentives as at the time of 'Boycott Chinese Products' has gained momentum with India being dependent on Chinese APIs for as much as 80%. MSMEs can play a major role in reviving the economy, but the government needs to give fiscal stimulus to the sector. E-commerce and hospitality have the power to recover sooner as they can provide big discounts and gain public faith by ensuring safety measures. The businesses have to evolve different leadership styles, changing ways of handling problems, following COVID guidelines while carrying on the routine operations. This chapter reflects the changed way of communication- a move from physical to digital, the communities evolving in handling the pandemic. The way of moving forward with relationships has changed, with some people struck alone has triggered mental issues, the plans are on a standby mode, etc. The pandemic is no doubt adding to the throes of life, but at the other end of the spectrum, there is something that we humans will learn after this phase is over.

Keywords: MSMEs, health, pharmaceutical, physical, digital

Introduction

"Coronavirus disease, more commonly known as Covid-19, is an infectious disease caused by a newly discovered coronavirus" (World Health Organization 2020) [1]. The global pervasiveness of covid-19 has designated the disease with the status of "Public Health Emergency," and it is acknowledged as a pandemic disease that does not consider any ethnic background and monetary level in both developed and developing economies. "The 2019 novel coronavirus epidemic expanded from Wuhan throughout China and is being exported to a growing number of countries, some of which have seen onward transmission." Preliminary attempts were focused on defining clinical pathways, identifying per acute patients, and curing the ailing, but later an imperative need of "public health activities" was encountered to explain the epidemiology of COVID-19 and describe its impact. Besides having a medical impact, COVID-19 also has an intense and consequential impact on the global economy. According to the World Economic Forum (2020), "Globally, the coronavirus shock is severe even compared to the Great Financial Crisis in 2007–08."

According to World Bank and World Health Organization (WHO), it was assessed the economic cost of COVID-19 to be between 2.2% to 4.8% of the global GDP (U.S. 3 trillion dollars) (Mukewar, 2020). In a recent article by Georgieva (2020), 1/3rd of the disease's economic cost will be direct, and the rest 2/3rd will be the indirect costs. While pondering about the economic costs of COVID-19, copious importance is employed on the direct and indirect costs of the disease. The direct cost represents the therapeutic intervention costs, and the indirect cost majorly focuses upon the costs due to productivity loss due to morbidity/mortality [2].

The pandemic's intangible costs are seldom brought into the consideration of the government, health agencies, and most importantly, amongst the people because it is complicated to quantify in a standardized manner. "Intangible costs are costs associated with pain, psychosocial suffering, changes in social functioning and activities of daily living caused by the disease" [3]. Therefore, the intangible costs of COVID-19 are substantial, and a diligent attempt is made to highlight the various intangible costs of COVID-19. In this chapter, we focused on the impact of COVID-19 on the Indian economy and the way forward.

COVID-19 and Micro Small and Medium Enterprises (MSME'S) in India

Micro Small and Medium Enterprises (MSMEs) are the major drivers of the Indian economy leading to inclusive development, boosting - demand, production, consumption, and employing millions of people in the country. The sector is staring at a bleak future due to COVID but still can open the doors to new opportunities. Everyone relies on the various strategies to be followed to get out from the worst of situations and help rebuild the sector.

There are 69 million micro, small and medium enterprises in India employing over 150 million people, and over 130 million people are self-employed [4]. Over 90% of all units fall in the micro category, distributed equally over rural and urban India, whereas small and medium ones are predominantly in urban India. Geographically, seven states alone account for 50% of all MSME's and these are Uttar Pradesh (14%), West Bengal (14%), Tamil Nadu (8%), Maharashtra (8%), Karnataka (6%), Bihar (5%) and Andhra Pradesh(5%) [5].

The sector was hit hard with the pandemic's onset as it forced the business operations to remain shut. The country and the economy were under the lockdown phase for almost five months which added to the sector's toll. The revenue loss to the sector was estimated at around Rs. Forty thousand crores a day, and more than 12 lakh crores during the lockdown [6]. Even during the unlock phase, only 30-40% of the MSMEs were opened up, hitting the sector hard. As a relief, the government came up with a guarantee-free loan, but the interest rate caused a major problem which hovered around 7.5% to 9.5%. However, again, the loan from the private sector banks and public sector banks differs on the interest rates, with some private lenders asking for 9.5% interest rates and only public banks giving it at around 7.5%, which is still much to be paid by those who are drowning [7].

It has been estimated that MSMEs recorded a downfall of minus 25.3 percent growth in net sales during Q1 FY21. A large number of small businesses had reduced their operations to negligible or temporarily shut down their operations due to a fall in demand and workers moved to their hometowns. As per a Crisil survey report, it was observed that MSMEs are staring at a steeper fall at 17-21 percent in their total revenues. According to government data, the registered MSMEs witnessed a growth of 18.49% in F.Y. 20 from F.Y. 19 [8]. Micro-enterprises dominate the MSME sector, according to the MSME Ministry data. They were registered the most as per segment-wise. Therefore, the growth that was seen in the number must have been at the same place as the number of units was shut down due to cash crunch during the pandemic period, taking the number somewhat back to where it was and hence adding to no growth in the aftermath period.

Another survey revealed that around 50% of MSMEs reported a decrease in order to them and an increase in inventories of raw materials and finished goods, along with a median 50% decline in income. Also, 50% of them reported a 20% increase in inventory inventories and finished goods each in quarter four due to the pandemic. Also, the supply chain was affected, and many jobs were lost in these industries due to the Coronavirus pandemic. In a sense, we can say that the package would not meet the losses already suffered by MSME.

The pandemic has created panic about the revival of growth in order to revive the economy. The government is doing the necessary things to revive the sector, but there are still loopholes. The credit funding scheme has been enrolled, but a major problem encountered with these units is that most of them are not registered anywhere as they are way too small, making it far impossible for the government to help them. The formal banking system supplies less than one-third (or about Rs. 11 lakh crores) of the credit they need, as most of the funding is done through the informal sector. Even if more liquidity is pushed, it has its threshold. Being out of the formal network, they did not feel the need to maintain the accounts, follow norms and regulations, pay taxes, etc., as it helps them bring their costs down. Nevertheless, it is important to map them at these times so that they can be pulled out of the situation. Many countries helped their smaller firms by providing wage subsidies directly, but this is not India's case because of the lack of mapping.

The loans to micro-units are sacrificed due to the bad debts created by the powerful bigger enterprises. This chapter focuses on how these units should be trusted with loans as they are drivers of the economy; loans should be offered without collateral or at lower rates of interest, as the case may be. A loan available at a cheaper rate of interest will drive the investors to take up the risks and invest further with an optimistic viewpoint. Additionally, it will somewhat help in promoting employment in the economy at this critical juncture. The step taken by the government regarding the credit line guarantee scheme is a major booster. According to a survey, only 22% of the MSMEs were aware of the scheme. So apparently, the awareness needs to be increased about such schemes, which is important.

This chapter stresses the diversification of the products which MSME produces, which at present stands at 6,000. These products are made cheaply, which can create demand for themselves. MSME's need to reinvent themselves according to the need of the hour, like producing masks, PPE kits, sanitizers, will help these products grow and mark their presence in the economy, and the "Vocal for Local" is bound to help them [9]. About 35% of MSMEs have shut down their businesses due to low chances of survival. Around 32% of MSMEs said it would take six months to recover, and 12% estimated the time at three months, according to the survey conducted by All India Manufacturers Organisation (AIMO).

Along with all the points mentioned above, another major factor is to be pointed out: ' payment.' The cash position of MSMEs needs to be studied well to take effective measures. Most of the MSMEs are micro-enterprises that do not receive their payments well on time. They operate on credit, so their cash positions remain precarious if the payment is delayed. Also, the delayed payment adds up to the delayed payment of salaries and raw materials, so there is a kind of cash cycle operating for the sector. According to the survey data, the payment supplies' time ranges from 90-180 days, making it a cumbersome process [10].

To contain them from shutting the operations, the government needs to provide them financial support and incentives. Safety measures should be introduced to feel free to return to work and resume production so that the supply chain can be restored [11].

As the rural part of the economy carries more potential with them, small industries should be promoted to fulfill the demand, and innovation and creativity should be taken hand to hand. It will also lead to more equitable distribution of wealth. The world is going digital these days; businesses should also be taken online. The goods and services produced should be promoted on digital platforms through MSME Sampark and MSME Sambandh [12]. Moreover, some success stories should also be promoted to gain consumers' trust, and people can come up with more innovative ideas to have built more MSMEs. Experts from various fields like economics and finance should be roped in to understand their problems and guide them to a new path. Technology can become the backbone of MSMEs in order to succeed in the post-COVID world. It was suggested that MSMEs use WhatsApp, Facebook, and other social media platforms to run their business in the post-COVID-19 situation. There is an immediate need for the partnerships of MSMEs with e-commerce players to target more customers. There is a need to organize digital trade fairs by the MSME to reach out to potential customers, suppliers, and lenders to grow their ecosystem and business. The entrepreneurs have started to stock easily accessible items that are high in demand among customers—almost 40% of MSME's increased safety and hygienic measures. The pandemic has also asserted many businesses to have tie-ups with digital e-commerce platforms to help make supplies of goods available to customers. Also, almost 60% of the enterprises reported a decline in their cash payments and going digital.

Also, steps should be taken to reduce the payment receiving time for the MSME sector, which almost stands at 90-180 days. The new normal has taken initiatives for itself by going digital. The payment can now be made digitally with just one click, which can somehow improve the situation. There is a dire need to provide alternate lending mechanisms for their revival. There is a need to continue monitoring the MSME's progress and design of fiscal stimulus to re-energize.

COVID-19 AND HEALTH AND PHARMACEUTICALS IN INDIA

The health and pharmaceutical sector plays a very vital role in the country. These sectors have been on their knees in the most developed countries, which have world-class facilities. This exposes the less developed countries to life-threatening risks where facilities are not up to the mark. Again, in less developed countries, the rural areas are most exposed to risk as the health facilities are minimal over there [13].

In India, the hospitals, especially government hospitals, are already in ICUs demanding oxygen of investment. The hospitals are struggling to keep up with sufficient staff in COVID designated hospitals, such as doctors, nurses, and ward boys, etc., as they are worried about their own lives. The state of civil hospitals in districts is really bad with toilets un-cleaned, bedsheets pilling up, etc. With Ministers infected with COVID and getting admitted to private hospitals exposes the unpreparedness of the government hospitals. The government should tweak its outlook towards fighting pandemics. Appropriate care should be given towards maintaining cleanliness in the hospitals; otherwise, people are at risk of getting infected with other infectious diseases.

Moreover, the patients and the people are dealing with mental health risks. The people during this time are left lonely with increasing mental health risks. 9% of the people in Japan, 22% of the USA, and 23% of the U.K. often feel lonely. Undoubtedly, in India, the joint family structure is prevalent, but COVID forced them to be alone. People are in quarantine facilities, and maintaining social distancing is the need of the hour [14, 15].

The sector saw operating losses of about Rs. 14,000-24,000 crores during the quarter. The private healthcare sector saw a drop of 70-80% in footfall test volumes. Private hospitals constitute more than 60% of beds at 8.5-9 lakhs, 60% of in-patients, and 80% of doctors in India [16].

COVID-19 AND DIGITALIZATION IN HEALTHCARE

Earlier, India's healthcare system required carrying bulging folders of medical reports, photocopies, blood test reports, etc., in hand when going to a doctor. The world has rolled out from a state of physical to digital. When everything is turning digital, the healthcare system is also in the race. There is an escalating use of artificial intelligence [17], robots in providing healthcare services, such as we saw the deployment of robots to take care of patients, provide medicines, etc., to avoid physical contact. It also provided an upper hand to prevent the spread of the virus [18, 19]. The pandemic forced the people to stay inside their homes due to the sudden attack of the virus. However, the companies responded well to the needs of the consumers by providing room for telemedicine. The patients were suffering due to the lack of medical and health advice. Some of the e-consultation apps such as Practo, Meddo, Doctor on Demand, etc. [20] saw an increase in their usage in recent times. These apps were in the market for a long time but gained importance during the pandemic. The apps provided the increased accessibility to medical advice through online video consultations and provided a digital prescription.

One of the major advantages of online consultation is people can reach out to doctors from remote locations. Also, when people are maintaining a social distance, these apps have come to the rescue. Even the contactless, online medicines deliveries are penetrating deep in the world. Apps have come up like PharmEasy, NetMeds, Practo, BookMeds, SmartMedics, WeChemist, etc. ensured the safe delivery of medicines at home. This chapter focuses on the digitization of healthcare systems, like creating Electronic Health Records. The data collected under this roof will not only be able to treat patients during the COVID time but can play a major role in the early detection of many diseases, can have a compiled record of patients' past medical history, immunizations, etc. and can help in providing effective treatment to them. The launch of the National Digital Health Blueprint (NDHB) by the government of India in 2019 to collect health data is a significant step towards digitalization in healthcare [21]. The countries are investing in digital healthcare data. A very good example is Israel, where the healthcare system has been paperless for almost 20 years.

COVID-19 AND PHARMA

The norms are being tweaked in the pharma sector in order to reduce the dependence on Chinese products. India imports around 63% or $3.4 billion worth of bulk drugs. India imports around 90% of its Active Pharmaceutical Ingredients (API's) and Key Starting Materials (KSM) from China. The government aspires to make India self-reliant to reduce China's dependence and give incentives to the companies to manufacture them. Providing them with production-linked incentives will help them to boost the manufacturing of 53 critical APIs. India has many drug and vaccine companies that are huge suppliers to the world, and its cost of manufacturing is 33% lower than that of the U.S., which should be taken as an opportunity to turn the countries of the world towards India to fulfill their demand [22].

The government's four schemes for developing bulk drugs and medical device parks in the country are bound to make India self-reliant in 8-10 years. The incentives worth 7,000 crores and grants to the tune of 1,000 crores are being given. The result is bound to yield results in the long term. Strict regulation and control should be ensured so that there is less risk to people's lives, as incidences of fake medicines, sanitizers, etc., are being popped up. Raids should take place, and punitive measures should be taken. During the pandemic, the prices of the raw materials have gone up, so, to gain market and be the major destination for other countries to be dependent on us, the prices need to be maintained at their competitive levels. There is uncertainty about the end of the pandemic, and the outcome of the scheme can not be found in the short term. India needs to identify its competency in the short term in maintaining prices to a low level, keeping manufacturing costs low, producing at a larger scale to grab the market, efficiently handling biowaste like disposing of them off in dustbins, collecting them, and disposing of them properly, preventing further harm [23].

Along with this, health records should be maintained of infections, their symptoms, the vulnerability of the disease, etc.; researchers have a hand-ready tool to research upon accordingly. The health level of the people of the country can easily be monitored through this. The development of vaccines and their procurement and distribution to the country's citizens also poses a major challenge to India's government. Many large-scale companies are in the process of making vaccines, and some are in the final stage, and some have even applied for emergency trials. In India, inoculating a major portion of the population is challenging. The government has already said that it will not go for complete immunization; rather, it will achieve herd immunity by giving vaccines to 60% of the population. Again the debatable question is about who is likely going to receive the vaccine first. According to the government, all health workers and front-line workers will be receiving vaccines taking the count to 300 million in the first phase. Afterward, the people aged 60 and above will be receiving vaccines. Nevertheless, shouldn't the people in the working-age group (who go out and bring viruses home) be vaccinated first?

Many rich countries have procured the coronavirus vaccine for their people to prevent them from spreading the virus. These countries can reach herd immunity by the end of 2021. Nevertheless, how the economically weaker countries are going to procure vaccines is a question. Britain, for example, approved the Pfizer vaccine for its people turning the game against the virus. Canada bought the most shots as each person can be vaccinated five times, considering the population's size.

In contrast, almost 70 economically weaker countries will only be able to vaccinate one in ten people; the world countries' heterogeneity is visible. No doubt, the WHO has backed a global vaccine program which is now known as COVAX-it ensures to provide for equitable distribution of COVID vaccines to economically weaker countries, and to date, 189 countries have become its members. However, the United States, not becoming its member, paints a different canvas. Even if COVAX delivers 2 billion doses by the end of 2021, it will represent only 20% of the countries' population that is part of the mechanism.

In developed nations, only 14-15% of the world population bought up around 55% of the vaccines so far. Nevertheless, and until the world is still optimistic about turning the tide against the virus that has now claimed nearly 1.5 million lives globally. The COVID-19 has provided opened various digital platforms to revamp the pharma sector's growth, such as industry's collaborations with physicians, virtual patient care 24/7, feedback on a real-time basis, etc. These digital avenues provide convenience and flexibility for all stakeholders. There is a need for the Indian pharma sector to adopt digitization and automation in its manufacturing and supply chain operations in the post-COVID era. After the post-COVID-19, the key drivers of the pharma sector's growth success will be technology, adequate finance, and competitiveness. Also, the domestic production of several medicines, medical equipment, raw material for pharmaceuticals needs to be ramped up to assist the economy both in growth and employment.

COVID-19 and Hospitality and Tourism in India

The hospitality industry is also keeping up itself with the latest trends. Everything from booking tickets to having access to breakfast meals on vacation is done digitally. Gone are the days when it was used to stand in line to book rail tickets or visit brick-and-mortar shops to a travel agent to book their trips. The processes have been improved and the customer experience enhanced with these trends. The hospitality industry's technology is allowing hotels to save costs and optimize experiences. For example, earlier, a well-decorated room, amazing service facilities, breakfast at your doorstep, a scenic view from the room was what defined the hospitality sector.

Nevertheless, the definition of new normal requires major changes in what it constitutes. Now people are more worried about their health and safety. The pandemic has created uncertainties about the sector as well as about the people employed in the sector. The sector employs four crores people, out of which 1.2 crores of people are expected to be laid off due to pandemic. The sector can revive earlier than expected if the safety levels are ensured. In hotels, delivering a feeling of safety, providing sanitizers, masks should be dispensed. The hoteliers are dispensing such technology, allowing them to control room lights and heating systems through apps, minimizing the need to touch buttons [24].

The post-COVID world will present a different picture altogether. During the hotel stay, the rooms should be equipped with only a set of essential items in order to avoid touch, providing packaged food, monitoring the number of people in the open spaces, say in the hotel, on the poolside, or in the cafeteria just by having technology in your pockets. The visitors can book their room prior, book their tables in advance in the cafeteria to avoid the rush, etc. Again, the A.I.-driven robots are the next biggest emerging trends deployed to perform complex and intelligent tasks. They deliver needful things to the room-avoiding physical contact with the hotel staff. The people's communication with the hotel staff can be done with voice recording and video recording as the situation demands. This chapter also focuses on the escalating digital trend of recognition technology, ranging from facial recognition to finger recognition.

Nevertheless, this is only used for reducing the time required for the payment process. So, it should be deployed to reduce human touch. Another major trend gaining around is virtual reality which can digitally transport people to a new place using 360-degree video. The hospitality industry can use it to provide a 360-degree view of the room, making customers informed about the room size, the essential items, the surrounding environment, etc., which is handy before the room booking. A person can visit the whole world sitting at their homes, according to their conveniences, at a very low cost. Nevertheless, experiencing reality is always different than what is experienced virtually [25].

Along with Virtual Reality, Augmented Reality also enhances real-world surroundings to the customers. This offers additional advantages to the customer providing them with graphical or informational overlays, local attractions, local areas, etc. Moreover, Artificial Intelligence can be deployed to answer customer questions or even at the reception and help desk area to improve response times and add to safety measures. Many online booking sites such as MakeMyTrip, Yatra, Goibibo, Expedia, Trip Advisor, etc., are creating wonderful experiences.

Digitalization is likely to determine the trend of modifying the sector to create the guests' experience as enjoyable as it was before COVID-19 [26]. Getting over this business is like a puzzle and putting together differently. The bond is bound to grow strong when safety is delivered.

Tourism is the largest service industry in India, worth $234 billion in 2018, the third-largest foreign exchange earner, contributing 9.2% to India's GDP in 2018 and supporting 42 million jobs which are 8.1% of total employment. The pandemic in force and the lockdown it triggered have disrupted the tourism sector very badly. The impact is direct because the movement of the people across the globe has been restricted. During April-June, the industry suffered a loss of Rs. 69,400 crores, and during the year, it is expected to suffer a loss of Rs. 1.25 trillion in the year 2020 [27]. Even when the lockdown procedures have eased and unlocked mode, people are not willing to step out of their homes. The fear of getting injected with the virus has entrenched in them. The outlook has to be changed to deal with the stressed sector.

A survey conducted by the Jones Lang LaSalle (JLL), Real Estate Consultancy Firm, has documented that 60 percent of the hotel operators felt that their hotel business could bounce back as of 2019 in terms of revenue a period of 13 to 24 months [28]. However, it was observed that 53 percent of the top hotel operators must shut down more than 80 percent of their operations as of the compulsory lockdown by the government. According to Confederation of Indian Industries (CII) and Hospitality Consulting Firm Hotelivate, "It was observed that the entire travel and tourism industry in India would incur a loss of Rs 5 lakh crore or $65.57 billion due to the current pandemic [29]. Furthermore, it was found that the organized segment will face a loss of $25 billion. It has been exhibited that the estimated revenue loss to travel agents and tour operators was $4.77 billion.

First of all, as the places are opening up, very few people are showing up. Along with that, mini lockdowns imposed by the states in the containment zones or imposing weekend lockdown or during the day's specific hours have exacerbated the situation. The situation has worsened with different states keeping different lockdowns or making compulsory quarantine. The flights have resumed their operations but are running with only 1/3rd of the capacity. Moreover, many countries are either putting up compulsory quarantine facilities or not allowing flights to carry on the operations, which is hampering the new normal. The countries are restricting travel to arrest the spread of the pandemic. Travel in the new normal requires a series of measures to revive the sector, including lifting the restrictions and gaining the travelers' confidence by ensuring safety and preventive measures. To the ones who are traveling, promoting health screening, and isolating those with any kind of symptoms, contact tracing people as soon as they report positive to limit the spread, take proper care of sanitation, and provide hygienic food to the travelers are some of the ways to fight. If traveling takes place between countries, testing should be made mandatory, and upon suspecting the cases, isolation should occur.

Coronavirus pandemic has given a clear indication that the tourism sector's success in the post-COVID-19 is based on accelerated digitalization and technological innovations. This chapter stresses the need to introduce new transportation processes, mobile applications, and automatic travel insurance plans for survival in the future.

COVID-19 and E-Education

The tables have turned upside down since the COVID-19 pandemic. The world is going through a change that it has never witnessed. The pandemic has created unprecedented challenges for the governments, administration, institutions, parents, and others to struggle for education. When every sphere of life is affected, each sector is bearing the toll; the education sector is no exception. The beginnings were rough when there was an instant shift to online teaching methods to compensate for the losses to some extent. According to UNESCO- "1.3 billion learners around the world were not able to attend school or university as of March 23, 2020," with 285 million young learners each in India [30]. E-learning or E-education became the buzzword of the year 2020. The schools, colleges, and Universities shifted to online devices to serve the educational purpose. It has made us realize that a lot many things can be done digitally, including education. Many online education delivery tart-ups emerged from nowhere to fulfill the needs like Udemy, Vedantu,

Eduauraa, Goodreads, etc. Many MOOC course providers like Coursera, Swayam, edx, Simplilearn, UpGrad, Open2Study, FutureLearn, etc., started providing easy access to a world-class education through online mode certificates after the completion of courses. They also partnered with many universities to provide online learning access free of cost or by providing financial aid. The future was at stake for many students, and they came to the rescue by providing an online master's degree program, P.G. diploma, Professional certification courses, etc., to adopt e-learning as a new normal.

Nevertheless, there are always two sides to the same coin. Society is striking a balance between the have and have nots. For many to go for online learning became a real challenge with lack of infrastructural facilities. The developed societies did not face much problem due to their sound infrastructural facilities, but in many developing societies where infrastructure building is still in progress, it is hard. Online education has its repercussions as it lacks the basic understanding and the classroom learning bond. The online shift was also challenging due to technical issues, students not having proper access to mobiles/laptops, etc. A study in India showed that during the lockdown, the sale of second-hand mobile phones, laptops doubled in India. A digital divide has been created where some have access to resources, and some do not. Specifically, the students from the rural areas are likely to bear the brunt of this pandemic as the technology has not penetrated deeply to all the students leading to inequality. So, the old chalk and duster method has been transformed into a modern way of online teaching.

Conclusion

The pandemic has put an economy's capabilities to the test. The world has caught a cold, and no doctor can prescribe a medicine for it. It has exposed the loopholes in the system which need to be considered. The virus has taken a toll on India, a country of 135 crores of people. The economy is crying for revival, and the sectors are screaming for funding.

It was noticed that the important outcome of the current pandemic is that it has brought the various stakeholders and government of the country to join hands in order to grow and to frame supportive policies in order to mitigate the various challenges created by the current pandemic. The economy can revive sooner than expected if a slew of measures is taken, keeping in mind the new normal. The major driver of Indian growth is India's MSME sector, which provides employment to lakhs of people and drives the growth rate. The sector needs formalization on a large scale so the government can provide that appropriate help at the right time, and the stressed units are funded well on time. Undoubtedly, India is a world leader in generics both domestically and internationally in the pharma sector, producing at a lower cost due to our comparative advantage but will take 8-10 years to be self-sufficient. So, the focus should be laid on reducing the cost of raw materials, products, etc.

Along with it, massive investment should be made in the workforce, equipment, beds, consumables, etc., to ensure the sector's preparedness. Safety is driving the world crazy these days. The same applies to hospitality and tourism as well. This new normal demand that rather than providing world-class or five-star facilities, providing safety services is going to take the business to new heights. Again, people should be made aware of the "Aarogya Setu" app. As of now, around 15 crores people are having the app installed on their phones, which is very less in a country of 135 crores people. We can get over this pandemic if proper measures are taken to contain the virus while opening the economy, on the other hand. Even when the vaccine arrives, proper care should be taken that the vaccine does not fall only in the rich's court; it should be provided to other people well in time. Mass immunization should be the goal of the government. Although it was observed that the government in India has taken various measures to curtail the adverse impact of the COVID-19 but still needs is to speed up the process of decision-making and implementation of the policies soon.

References

[1] "Coronavirus 2020." *World Health Organization.* Available from: https://www.who.int/health-topics/coronavirus#tab=tab_1.

[2] "The IMF explains the economic lessons from China's fight against coronavirus. 2020." *World Economic Forum.* Available from: https://www.weforum.org/agenda/2020/03/imf-economic-lessons-from-china-fight-against-coronavirus/.

[3] "Potential impact of the COVID-19 epidemic: what we know and what we can do"; *International Monetary Fund 2020*; Available from: https://blogs.imf.org/2020/03/04/potential-impact-of-the-coronavirus-epidemic-what-we-know-and-what-we-can-do/.

[4] Pramanik, Ayan. 2020. "A quarter of MSMEs may shut shop if the lockdown persists," *The Economic Times*. March 30. Accessed September 15.

[5] https://economictimes.indiatimes.com/small-biz/sme-sector/a-quarter-of-msmes-may-shut-shop-if-the-lockdown-persists/articleshow/74880940.cms?from=mdr.

[6] Mishra, Udit. 2020. "Explained: Why are Medium, Small, Micro Enterprises worst hit by Covid-19 lockdown?" *The Indian Express*. May 7. Accessed October 26. https://indianexpress.com/article/explained/coronavirus-india-lockdown-msme-sector-crisis-government-relief-package-6395731/.

[7] Kaur, Gurneel. 2020. "Revenue Loss of MSMEs Estimated at More Than 12 Lakh Crore Since Lockdown," *Grain Mart India*. May 13. Accessed September 17. https://www.grainmart.in/news/revenue-loss-of-msmes-estimated-at-more-than-12-lakh-crore-since-lockdown/.

[8] Roy Suhita. 2020. "Only 30-40% MSME units have opened for work in Unlock Phase 1: FISME's Animesh Saxena." *Economic Times*. June 18. Accessed September 19. https://economictimes.indiatimes.com/small-biz/sme-sector/only-30-to-40-msme-units-have-opened-for-work-in-unlock-phase-1-fismes-animesh-saxena/articleshow/76418627.cms.

[9] Soni, Sandeep. 2020. "India's MSME sector swells, adds these many enterprises in FY20; micro businesses dominate." *Financial Express*. March 23. Accessed November 10. https://www.financial express.com/industry/sme/msme-other-indias-msme-sector-swells-adds-these-many-enterprises-in-fy20-micro-businesses-dominate/1906979/.

[10] Rastogi, Vasundhara. 2020. "Micro, Small, and Medium Enterprises in India – An Explainer," *India Briefing*. May 14.Accessed September 22. https://www.india-briefing.com/news/micro-small-medium-enterprises-india-explainer-17887.html/#:~:text=As%20per%20the%20official%20estimates,total%20MSMEs%20in%20the%20country.

[11] Mehrotra et al. 2020. "Impact of COVID-19 pandemic on micro, small and medium enterprises (MSME's)." *India Report, Microave Consulting*. June. Accessed October 29. https://www.microsave.net/2020/06/04/impact-of-covid-19-pandemic-on-micro-small-and-medium-enterprises-msmes-india-report/.

[12] Nishtha Saluja. 2020. "Over one-third MSMEs start shutting shop as recovery amid Covid-19 looks unlikely: AIMO survey." *The Economic Times Rise*. June 2. Accessed November 3.

[13] https://economictimes.indiatimes.com/small-biz/sme-sector/over-one-third-msmes-start-shutting-shop-as-recovery-amid-covid-19-looks-unlikely-aimo-survey/articleshow/76141969.cms?from=mdr.

[14] "MSME – The growth engine of New India." 2020. *Make in India*. August. Accessed October 17. https://www.makeinindia.com/msme.

[15] Ling, G. H., H. O., C. M. 2020. "Effects of the Coronavirus (COVID-19) Pandemic on Social Behavior's: from a Social Silemma Perspective." *Technium Social Sciences Journal* 25; 7(1):312-20.

[16] Wilder, S. A., Freedman, D. O. 2020. "Isolation, Quarantine, Social Distancing and Community Containment: Pivotal Role for Old-style Public Health Measures in the Novel Coronavirus (COVID-19) Outbreak." *Journal of Travel Medicine* 27(2): 1-20.

[17] *Social Distancing in the Time of COVID-19: the Hidden Cost? Mental Health, Outlook. 2020*; Available from: https://www.outlookindia.com/website/story/opinion-social-distancing-in-the-time-of-covid-19-the-hidden-cost-mental-health/354748.

[18] "COVID-19 leaves private healthcare sector in financial distress: FICCI-EY study." 2020. *Business Line, The Hindu*. April 17. https://www.thehindubusinessline.com/economy/macro-economy/covid-19-leaves-private-healthcare-sector-in-financial-distress-ficci-ey-study/article31362331.ece\\Accessed September 2020.

[19] Agrawal Akshat, Rajesh Arora, Ranjna Arora, Prateek Agrawal. (2021). Applications of Artificial Intelligence and Internet of Things for Detection and Future Directions to Fight against COVID-19. In edited book on *Emerging Technologies for Battling Covid-19,* pp. 107-119, Springer.

[20] Agrawal Prateek, Vishu Madaan, Aditya Roy, Rajani Kumari & Harshal Deore. (2021). FOCOMO: Forecasting and monitoring the worldwide spread of COVID-19 using machine learning methods, *Journal of Interdisciplinary Mathematics,* pp. 1-25. doi: 10.1080/09720502.2021.1885812.

[21] Madaan, V, A Roy, C Gupta, P Agrawal, A Sharma, C Bologa, R Prodan. (2021). XCOVNet: Chest X-ray Image Classification for COVID-19 Early Detection Using Convolutional Neural Networks. *New Generation Computing,* pp. 1-15, 2021. doi: 10.1007/s00354-021-00121-7.

[22] Awasthi Prashasti. 2020. "Some popular telemedicine apps for e-consultation." *The Hindu Business Line*. June 5. Accessed November 9. https://www.thehindubusinessline.com/info-tech/some-popular-telemedicine-apps-for-e-consultation/article31754671.ece.

[23] Mabiyan Rashmi. 2020. "India bullish on A.I. in healthcare without electronic health records." *Economic Times. India Times*. January 6. Accessed December 5. https://health.economictimes.indiatimes.com/news/health-it/india-bullish-on-ai-in-healthcare-without-ehr/73118990.

[24] Narula, Sandeep. 2020. "Impact of coronavirus on future of Indian pharma sector." *PharmaBiz*. May 29. Accessed September 9.

http://www.pharmabiz.com/ArticleDetails.aspx?aid=126457&sid=9.

[25] Dadhich, Abhishek. 2020. "The COVID-19 pandemic and the Indian pharmaceutical industry." *European Pharmaceutical Review."* April 22. Accessed September 8. https://www.europeanpharmaceuticalreview.com/article/117413/the-covid-19-pandemic-and-the-indian-pharmaceutical-industry/#:~:text=The%20impact%20of%20the%20SARS,shortages%20in%20China's%20manufacturing %20plants.

[26] Pandya Maulik. 2018. "How Digitalization Transformed Old Trends of Hospitality and Tourism Industry." *Evince Development Blog.* October 24. https://evincedev.com/blog/how-digitalization-transformed-old-trends-of-hospitality-and-tourism-industry/#:~:text=Data%20plays%20an%20important%20role,the%20payment%20for%20the%20same.&text=They%20use%20customer%20data%20to,restricting%20to%20avail%20the%20services.

[27] "Key Digital Trends in the Hospitality Industry." *Revfine Optimising Revenue*. https://www.revfine.com/digital-trends-hospitality-industry/.

[28] Ristova C., Dimitrov N. 2019. "Digitalization in the Hospitality Industry: Trends That Might Shape The Next Stay Of Guests." *International Journal of Information, Business and Management*, Vol. 11, No.3, 2019. https://search.proquest.com/openview/dd782934aadd3a22bb13fb60542c617c/1?pq-origsite=gscholar&cbl=2032142.

[29] Dash, Jayajit. 2020. "Covid-19 impact: Tourism industry to incur Rs 1.25 trillion revenue loss in 2020," *Business Standard*. April 28. Accessed October 5. https://www.business-standard.com/article/economy-policy/covid-19-impact-tourism-industry-to-incur-rs-1-25-trn-revenue-loss-in-2020-120042801287_1.html.

[30] "Coronavirus impact: 60% hotel operators feel revenue recovery to take 2 years." 2020. *Business Today*. July 1. Accessed December 11. https://www.businesstoday.in/current/corporate/coronavirus-impact-60-per-cent-hotel-operators-expect-two-year-revenue-recovery-period-hospitality-industry/story/408594.html.

[31] "Travel and tourism sector likely to lose Rs. 5 lakh crore due to COVID-19 crisis: Report." 2020. *Economic Times*. September 9. Accessed October 2. https://economictimes.indiatimes.com/industry/services/travel/travel-and-tourism-sector-likely-to-lose-rs-5-lakh-crore-due-to-covid-19-crisis-report/articleshow/78015214.cms.

[32] McCarthy N. 2020. "COVID-19's Staggering Impact on Global Education." *World Economic Forum.* March 26. Accessed December 1. https://www.weforum.org/agenda/2020/03/infographic-covid19-coronavirus-impact-global-education-health-schools/.

SECTION 4. LIFE AFTER COVID-19

In: Impacts and Implications of COVID-19 ISBN: 978-1-53619-670-2
Editors: Anand Sharma et al.

Chapter 9

POTENTIAL NATURAL RESOURCES FOR AGRICULTURE RESEARCH IN INDIA DURING COVID-19 PANDEMIC

S. Azhagu Madhavan[1,*], P. Vinotha[2], V. Uma[2] and M. Mahadevi[3]
[1]PG & Research Department of Zoology & Biotechnology, A Veeriya Vandayar Memorial Sri Pushpam College, Poondi, Thanjavur, Tamil Nadu, India
[2]PG & Research Department of Bio-Chemistry, Bharathidasan University, Tiruchirappalli, Tamilnadu, India
[3]PG & Research Department of Botany & Microbiology, A Veeriya Vandayar Memorial Sri Pushpam College, Poondi, Thanjavur, Tamil Nadu, India

ABSTRACT

The lockdown measures duration led us to consider how potential food crops and agriculture play a vital role in this pandemic

* Corresponding Author's E-mail: mathavan062@gmail.com.

situation. Except for the Health services and essential services, the agriculture sector plays a significant role in feeding the country's large population. (COVID – 19) pandemic crises and prompts changes in paddy cultivation. At first, we study the role of paddy cultivation for human beings in the lockdown scenario, and a second, it entirely covered the farmers and their challenges during paddy cultivation in the lockdown period. Also, it elaborates on their input access, labor facilities in this situation (Human Resources), market availability, and these supply chain for paddy then its by-products. Also, it Prompts Changes in Paddy Cultivation. Finally, the study carried about the dynamic usage of paddy by-products to improve the standard of living of the farmers, which means mushroom cultivation, vermicomposting, ropes, packing material, pellets, paper making, mulching techniques, animal feeding, rice bran wax, industrial-grade crude oil, husk briquettes and also it acts as a carrier for biofertilizers organisms.

Year by year, the risks faced by Indian farmers keep aggravating in terms of low rainfall, price volatility, and rising debts. However, the global pandemic risks of COVID-19 have posed new challenges in the agriculture sector that is already under threat. The harvesting of rabi crops was at stake with the nationwide lockdown that coincided with creating a shortage of both labor and equipment. It creates an urgent need to devise some sustainable and practical strategies to mitigate the problems occurring at the farm gate level.

Keywords: COVID-19, biofertilizers, agriculture, food security, biosaline agriculture

INTRODUCTION

Coronavirus has impacted the world's food supply chains and economies. It has added to an immediate effect on individuals' everyday exercises, intruding on the admission of solid and suitable food. People are needed to buy vegetables in more significant amounts. The pay of families subject to everyday compensation has been diminished, which will, in general, build people's food insecurity. Similarly, the COVID-19 pandemic has majorly affected both the creation and utilization of agrarian items because of the absence of agri-inputs. Moreover, the absence of work in the lockdown has influenced the collecting, planting, and relocating of paddy, which decreased the yield. Business ranchers confronting troubles in selling their merchandise and homestead items are frequently squandered and spoiled on the field [1]. An irreparable loss of development around the globe has been set off by the COVID-19 pandemic. Meanwhile, different areas of wellbeing, schooling, farming, the travel industry, and framework have been influenced by the pandemic. In India, poor people and everyday breadwinners are generally influenced and defenseless. The agrarian item areas are additionally influenced in light of the fact that the inventory of work that works consistently is genuinely hampered. In such an emergency, during a delayed lockdown and disturbance of the food framework, it is significant for an individual to assemble a versatile ability to adjust to the developing setting and keep up the current food framework [2-7]. The COVID-19 pandemic has prompted outrageous and worldwide human medical conditions [8-10]. Required countermeasures against the infection, for example, controls and different limitations, will persevere basically for a while with muddled end dates. By confining human development, worldwide endeavors to control the infection at last causes monetary stuns that can affect the tasks of cultivating and food frameworks worldwide. We are, as of now, seeing the indirect impacts of the CoVID-19 pandemic on horticulture and unified exercises across the globe. Quarantine mediations significantly affect the inventory of work for critical time-ranch exercises, from planting vegetable yields to organic product gathering. As the emergency advances, these effects are probably going to turn out to be broader and profoundly felt in the horticultural areas and public economies [3]. The centrality and seriousness of the pandemic, and its possible effect on agribusiness around the world, call for pleasing appearance in both the short and long terms. The immediate ramifications for the worldwide organization of food and horticultural frameworks on which we depend so vigorously should be figured out. We should screen startling dangers, weaknesses, and fundamental changes to consider transient impacts just as those that might be enduring or irreversible [11]. In this part, we examined the impact of the lockdown of COVID-19 on Indian horticulture and farming examination.

EFFECT OF COVID-19 ON AGRICULTURE

Quite possibly the vastest and ground-breaking area in the food security of the nation is the farming area [12]. The evolved way of life is a significant organization, and farming is quite possibly the central part of the nation. Food handling, the stock of crude materials to different businesses, occupations, and the age of pay are among the prior administrations of the rural area [13-15]. In the accompanying areas, we examined the effect of COVID19 on various parts of horticulture.

Food Security

India is the country that has the most significant number of individuals overall who do not get enough food to eat. The latest yearning pervasiveness figures are in India for 2011-12 portrayed that 47.2 crore individuals in India were not acquired the base measure of food required for them to carry on with a good life [16]. FAO food weakness review gauges uncovered that the number of people confronting moderate to extraordinary food frailty in India expanded from 36 crores in 2014-15 to 45 crores in 2017-1919. Food request has been affected by a decrease in deals and purchasing power [17]. Froze clients are accumulating food, which thusly has impacted the inventory and cost of food [18]. Food weakness may happen because of the decrease in worldwide exchange, interruptions in the food supply chain, and food creation. The interruption of food frameworks and the impact on food security is a pressing concern. Food dispersion networks have been altogether disturbed across the pay continuum in practically all countries, with substantial negative impacts for the most hindered.

Creative Saline Agriculture

Probably the most effortless approach to handle the saltiness issue while intending to create safe harvest plants for numerous pressure factors is to utilize halophytes that can make due in seawater salt focuses [19]. The development of salt-open-minded harvest plants does not ensure the expulsion of salt from the dirt. They just endure saltiness stress to the most excellent aspect their capacity; nonetheless, halophytes can eliminate the salt, and they can be utilized for development with horticultural plants, or they can be developed ahead of time of the development of rural yield plants to eliminate the salt by collecting in their organelles [20]. Modestly or profoundly saline soils would then be able to be remediated through the utilization of halophytes, and these specks of dirt can be remembered for agrarian regions in a practical way.

Biosaline Agriculture

Saline farming is a solid option for the fate of horticulture. The expansion in supplement interest and arriving at freshwater is a significant test. Under these conditions, saline horticulture has an arising role [21]. It creates explicit trimming frameworks for saline conditions, using the limit of specific plants to develop under saline conditions alongside the utilization of saline soil and water assets with improved soil and water the board techniques.

Parts of Saline Agriculture

Salt-lenient plants and halophytes in different saline conditions and improve their efficiency by plant rearing and agronomics [22]. Utilization of saline soils by inventive administration rehearses for crop creation. The saltiness in different saline climates through progress in the foundation for the water system and sewage adjusted to the requirements of explicit salt open-minded and halophytic crops.

Biofertilizers

These potential natural manures would assume an essential job in maintainability and efficiency of soil and furthermore ensure the climate as eco-friendly and savvy contributions for the ranchers. They are a savvy, eco-friendly, and inexhaustible wellspring of plant supplements to enhance substance composts in a manageable rural framework. Biofertilizer, an elective wellspring of N-compost, particularly rhizobia in beneficial vegetable interaction, is a setup innovation [23]. The utilization of biofertilizers can likewise forestall the consumption of the natural dirt issue. From a broad perspective, the term can be utilized to incorporate all-natural assets utilized for plant development that become accessible for take-up by plants through microorganisms or plant affiliations or collaborations. The information on applied microbial inocula has a long history that is passed from age to age of ranchers. It began with limited scope fertilizer cultivating which has clearly shown biofertilizer capacity. This was perceived when the deterioration of natural deposits and agrarian results expanded, and a solid yield collection was acquired. Biofertilizers are regularly seen as more costly than the compound manures because of the absence of abilities and innovation in their creation from reasonable and squander substrates. Plus, their impact on the harvests is delayed when contrasted with compound manures [24]. Special consideration is needed in their stockpiling and bundling. Fair treatment of microbial inocula is required with the goal that they stay compelling for broadened use. As biofertilizers are plans containing living life forms, their proficiency relies upon natural conditions [25, 26]. Subsequently, results of the utilization of biofertilizers will undoubtedly be conflicting. Because of various human exercises, the climate is the most influenced. In like manner, agrarian exercises have assumed an inexorably prominent position since the approach of human-made synthetic substances such as fertilizers, pesticides, and growth regulators to meet the need of a never-developing population. Chemical manures in the present moment can be very valuable in the harvest creation; however in since a long time ago run they are only causing harm to humans and to the typical flora of the soil. It antagonistically bestows the impact of soil fruitfulness [27].

In the event that we can eliminate the chemical fertilizers utilization and rely on more environmentally friendly methods like changing to biofertilizer for the same, we caner store the fertility of the soil and thus can improve the growth of harvests without destructing the natural habitat of the dirt that is responsible for growth and development of plants. Biofertilizers are the misleadingly prepared microbial inoculants of different a strain that helps upgrading the take-up of nutrients by plants and enhances the quality of soil by their association in the rhizosphere [28]. When applied either on the topsoil or through seed vaccinations, they upgrade the development of plants and developing soil microflora.

Results and Discussion

Difficulties and Possibilities of COVID-19 in Agriculture

Amidst COVID-19, as a worldwide pandemic, there were not many chances rising up out of the rural emergency. Since individuals are kept to remaining at home, and there is a deficiency of overabundance nutritious vegetables, the thought and association of a person in-home nursery and housetop cultivating has been advancing. Cultivating exercises for the planting of blossoms and vegetables have become highly significant where all individuals from the family are effectively involved. Likewise, the pertinence of means cultivating has emerged [20]. The people group way to deal with cultivating was a critical feature during the lockdown as there was no need for ranchers who develop vegetables on a limited scale. To get a reasonable cost available, either an individual necessity to deliver an immense measure of vegetables or enter different gatherings. The distributer would quit stacking the more modest volume of production despite the fact that the transportation has been made adaptable. Also, during an emergency, dried vegetables could be one of the decisions to forestall the deficiency of vegetables in the district [14]. The dried results of mushrooms and vegetables are profoundly primary and organized. It has been found in domesticated animals that milk can be changed over into milk items like margarine, ghee, cheddar, curd, cheese, and paneer. There was a lack of work to complete horticultural work on the homestead because of COVID-19, as there was trouble in the accessibility of work during the collecting of the standing harvests. Be that as it may, this has opened the entryway for an automation approach in the great rural area, where hardware parts can be utilized in appropriate zones with more enormous hectares of land to do agrarian exercises, for example, seed planting and yield reaping. Because of the absence of item supply, the importance of the nearby food accessible in the town or local location has been felt by individuals [20, 25]. Individuals were keener on eating nearby nourishments as they are more nutritious instead of attempting to search for extemporized things. Individuals have begun offering need to the nearby seeds accessible in their general vicinity, in any event, for the development of yields. Somewhat, they have utilized the seeds they have saved in their homes. The utilization of nearby and native products has expanded, prompting a person's independence.

Enhanced Income for Rural Poor

Today, it has been a great challenge to provide safe, healthy, and nutritious food for poor income groups and the undernourished population of the developing world to sustain and lead a healthy life. The ever-rising cost, shortage, and unreliable supply of healthy food in the developing and underdeveloped countries have resulted in the search for cheap and alternative sources of healthy and nutritious food, and the wild species of edible plants have been identified as a potential source of nutrition [7]. To supplement the nutritional requirement with dietary diversification from such plant species, the demand from consumers in developing countries is growing, which provides the opportunity to exploit the untapped potential of wild edibles for domestication. The systematic cultivation with the development of agro-techniques for such non-conventional plants may prove to be rewarding and will ultimately create new market niches for these crops [3, 21]. These market opportunities can provide livelihood options and generate additional income for the rural populace in less-favored environments where these crops have comparative advantages over major staples or commercial crops.

Ecosystem Stability

Climate change has been perceived as a serious threat and will have a significant impact on agriculture due to erratic rainfall, more demands for water, and enhanced biotic and abiotic stresses. The increase in temperature will have a more significant effect on reproductive biology, and the reduction in water could be detrimental to crop productivity. The changes in climate and the degradation of land and water resources have led to a growing interest in the search for new crops and species that are adapted to challenging environments such as poor soil or degraded vegetation [18]. These challenges could be addressed through the identification of potential wild edible plant species which are easy to grow, hardy in nature and can tolerate high temperature, withstand flood, drought, salinity, and can use nutrients and water efficiently.

Impact of COVID-19 on Agriculture and Agricultural Research in India

Information and Communication Technology (ICT) has been recognized as a significant way of connecting farmers' produce to the markets. Because of the lockdown, the transportation of goods has been affected. However, few of the farmers' production processing initiatives have been identified and sold through ICT tools.ICT tools are becoming essential in crisis situations [14]. Different media have been used where farmers post their products on social media and are contacted by interested people and receive the products at home. This has generated an understanding that ICT can be a successful alternative to selling and educating individuals about farmers' goods. Similarly, it would be good to use ICT resources to link up with agricultural experts and extension staff to bring about revolutionary changes in agriculture.

Microbial Pigments: Future Route for Public Health and Environment

Natural pigment origination from microbial sources (bacteria, fungi, and microalgae) as secondary metabolites is found to be more valuable and demandable than synthetic pigments. Microbial pigments have economic potential and industrial importance, providing opportunities for application in textile, pharmaceutical, food, and cosmetics. However, their current volume of production still has not attained the optimum level to satisfy the demand aroused due to the recent awareness for natural products [25]. The current novel strategies like gene-splicing, molecular biology techniques, and fermentation technologies are highly contributing to the maximum yield of bacterial pigments. Nowadays, it is becoming more popular because of not forming harmful intermediates and thereby protecting both environment and humans.

Summary and Conclusion

Crop Production and Availability of Seeds and Fertilizers

The labor, logistics, harvesting machinery, and plants are not operating at maximum levels till now. A lot of the migrant workers were headed back home, thereby creating problems for farms, seed production areas, seed packing, and crop harvesting [5]. This is the concern for all companies and stakeholders across India. The impact of the Covid-19 pandemic on Indian fertilizer production capacity has been widespread and facing logistical constraints due to movement restrictions, road closures, lack of enough truck drivers to make deliveries, labor shortage at the production plant, limited human resources, limited storage capacity resulting in pressure on the evacuation of materials, low availability of raw materials and consumable materials- bag, chemicals, and government restrictions and protocols.

Food Production and Distribution

Most of the countries have taken procedures such as travel bans, home confinement, and business restrictions to control infection rates. Farmers are compelled to hold their unsold produce for a more extended period of time due to the perishable nature of Agriculture produce. This has led to a reduction in food quality as well as an increase in the cost of cultivation.

Livestock Sector

The livestock production sector, segmented by type into dairy, meat, poultry, aquaculture, and others, is affected significantly due to the increased rate of virus spread. Regional demand for chicken, mutton, and fish are decreased, and basic food or essentials have been on the rise. Market growth has also affected due to the shutdowns of the food chain services, including restaurants. Despite the high demand for meat, aquaculture, and dairy products amidst the coronavirus, the supply chain has witnessed a host of disruption, which is stopping producers from providing their products in the market. Disruptions in the supply chains are causing wastage of fresh produce even though there are a high demand and food shortage for dairy produce. The impact under consumers of the pandemic will humidify the requirement for animal protein, subsequently affecting the feed market.

Labour

Rural laborers in India, absence of appropriate wellbeing administrations and social security because of practically zero investment funds. During the COVID-19 pandemic, numerous casual farming laborers are committing to work for their food, notwithstanding the self separation convention. On account of the non-accessibility of work, hurt activities in numerous parts. Costs of farming items have fallen because of ascending in labor expenses and absence of access.

Shortage of Public Goods

Making the food grains, products of the soil, and other fundamental things accessible to customers, both in metropolitan and provincial regions, is the most basic test. In different nations around the globe, the Covid-19 pandemic is spreading at different rates. Considering these difficulties, the worldwide economy is going through a new and diverse experience that is presently occurring in various nations [1, 26]. The cultivating area was not impervious to the financial mischief brought about by the episode and experienced extreme damage. If the necessary strides for practical creation in farming and the protection of the pattern of market interest are not taken, wellbeing and food security will confront an emergency. In spite of gigantic human misfortunes affecting various enterprises around the world, an individual can at present see the silver covering that can come over because of COVID-19 with the elevating of lockdown. To save independence, each degree of government ought to be more connected with farming exercises. Sanitation and wholesome security are essential to the human, social and financial turn of events [20]. The prosperity of a nation is directly linked with the health and happiness of the people, and a country could only be secured if the citizens have access to healthy food to meet their nutritional needs for a healthy life. However, access to nutritious food continues to be a significant concern in developing countries; millions of people continue to suffer from malnutrition, which is a cause for various kinds of diseases and premature death of children and women. In this perspective, the wild edible plants embedded with rich nutrient potentials have emerged as the best option not only to provide required nutrients but also to enhance the availability of healthy and nutritious food. These plants have sustained human populations as a source of food, livelihoods, health, and culture. They are vital biological assets for the rural poor and can help improve the overall welfare of millions of tribal populations across the globe. The potential of WEPs in generating income and livelihood options for rural masses has been acknowledged around the world. The high cost, shortage, and inadequate supply of nutritious food for the malnourished population of developing countries create market opportunities for these food plants to satisfy their dietary sufficiency and nutritional adequacy. Despite the vast potential and recognized importance, the wild plant species have remained underutilized and underexplored, and subsequently, this valuable plant wealth and their potential habitats have gradually waned. The erosion of these plant resources can have immediate consequences on nutritional security and the welfare of the poor. Therefore, emphasis on the conservation, evaluation, and utilization of these novelties is the acknowledgment of the need for attaining food and nutrition security and sustainable socio-economic growth. Likewise, it has been expected that a significant number of travelers would re-visitation farming and become included. Consequently, considering the COVID-19 emergency in India, legitimate strategies, spending designation, appropriations on data sources, merchandise, and ensured markets are destined to see a transformation in horticulture.

ACKNOWLEDGMENTS

We would like to express our sincerest condolences to the patients and families who suffered from the COVID-19 outbreak. We also greatly appreciate the healthcare personnel and staff members who worked together to overcome the COVID-19 outbreak.

REFERENCES

[1] World Health Organization. Coronavirus disease COVID-19). (2019). *Pandemic.* Available from: https://www.who.int/emergencies/diseases/novel-coronavirus-, accessed on August 27, 2020.

[2] Ministry of Health and Family Welfare, Government of India. *COVID-19 cases in India.* (2020) on August 27, Available from https://www.mohfw. gov.in, accessed.

[3] U.S. National Library of Medicine. *ClinicalTrials.gov.* (2020). On June 27, Available from: https://clinicaltrials.gov/, accessed.

[4] *World Health Organization. Draft landscape of COVID-19 candidate vaccines.* (2020), on August 27. Available from: https://www.who.int/.publications/m/item/draft-landscape-of-covid-19 candidate vaccines, accessed.

[5] Directorate General of Health Services, Ministry of Health and Family Welfare, Government of India. *Clinical management protocol: COVID-19. (2020) on June 27, 2020.* Available from: https://www.mohfw.gov.in/pdf/ClinicalManagementProtocolfor COVID19.pdf, accessed.

[6] *Approval of Favipiravir tablets to Glenmark Pharmaceuticals and Remdesivir injection to Cipla Ltd, Hetero Drugs and Mylan Labs.* (2020) on August 27, Available from: https://cdsco.gov.in/ opencms/pencms/system/modules/CDSCO.WEB/elements/downl oad_ file_division.jsp?num_id=NjIxMw.

[7] National Institutes of Health. *Coronavirus disease 2019 (COVID-19) treatment guidelines.* (2020) accessed on June 27, Available from: https:// covid19treatmentguidelines.nih.gov/.

[8] Agrawal, Akshat, Rajesh Arora, Ranjna Arora, Prateek Agrawal. (2021). Applications of Artificial Intelligence and Internet of Things for Detection and Future Directions to Fight against COVID-19. In edited book on *Emerging Technologies for Battling Covid-19,* pp. 107-119, Springer. Prateek Agrawal, Vishu Madaan, Aditya Roy, Rajani Kumari & Harshal Deore. (2021).

[9] FOCOMO: Forecasting and monitoring the worldwide spread of COVID-19 using machine learning methods, *Journal of Interdisciplinary Mathematics,* pp. 1-25. doi:10.1080/09720502. 2021.1885812.

[10] Madaan, V, A Roy, C Gupta, P Agrawal, A Sharma, C Bologa, R Prodan. (2021). XCOVNet: Chest X-ray Image Classification for COVID-19 Early Detection Using Convolutional Neural Networks. *New Generation Computing,* pp. 1-15, 2021. doi:10.1007/s00354 -021-00121-7.

[11] Arnold, SL, and F Buckner. (2020).Hydroxychloroquine for treatment of SARS-CoV-2 infection? Improving our confidence in a model-based approach to dose selection. *Clin Transl Sci;* 13: 642-5.

[12] Smit, C, MYM Peeters, JN van den Anker, CA Knibbe. (2020). Chloroquine for SARS-CoV-2: Implications of Its unique pharmacokinetic and safety properties. *Clin Pharmacokinet;* 59: 659-69.

[13] Zhang, GQ, C Hu, Lj, Luo, F, Fang, YF, Chen, JG Li, Zy Peng, and H Pan, (2020). Clinical Features and Treatment of 221 Patients with COVID-19 in Wuhan, China. *SSRN Electronic Journal.* https://doi.org/10.2139/ssrn.3546095.

[14] Madhavan, S Azhagu, P Vinotha, V Uma, S Ganesan & J Senthil. (2020). COVID-19 therapeutic and prevention aminoquinolines against coronavirus disease (COVID-19): chloroquine or hydroxychloroquine review. *International Journal of Indian Psychology,* 8(3), 1162-1169. DIP:18.01.121/20200803, doi: 10.25215/0803.121.

[15] Sohrabi, C, Z Alsafi, N O'Neill, M, Khan, A, Kerwan, A, Al-Jabir, C, Iosifidis, and R, Agha. (2020). World Health Organization Declares Global Emergency: A Review of the 2019 Novel Coronavirus (COVID-19). *International Journal of Surgery.* 76 (February): 71–76. https://doi.org/10.1016/j.ijsu.2020.02.034.

[16] Rothan, HA, and SN Byrareddy, (2020). The Epidemiology and Pathogenesis of Coronavirus Disease (COVID-19) Outbreak. *Journal of Autoimmunity.* 109 (February): 102433. https://doi.org/10.1016/j.jaut.2020.102433.

[17] Zhang, J, M Litvinova, Y Liang, Y Wang, W Wang, S Zhao. (2020). Changes in contact patterns shape the dynamics of the COVID-19 outbreak in China. *Science;* 368 1481-6.

[18] Choudhary, ML, V Vipat, S Jadhav, A Basu, S Cherian, P Abraham, (2020). Development of in vitro transcribed RNA as positive control for laboratory diagnosis of SARS-CoV-2 in India. *Indian J Med Res;* 151: 251-4.

[19] Tomasi, D, (2020). Coronavirus Disease (COVID-19). *A Socio-epidemiological Review.* Vermont Academy of Arts and Sciences. 1: 1-7.

[20] Gupta N, S Agrawal, P Ish, S Mishra, R Gaind, G Usha. (2020). Clinical and epidemiologic profile of the initial COVID-19 patients at a tertiary care centre in India. *Monaldi Arch Chest Dis;* 10: 90.

[21] Dong, Y, X Mo, Y Hu, X Qi, F Jiang, Z Jiang. (2020). Epidemiology of COVID-19 among children in China. *Pediatrics;* 145: e20200702.

[22] U.S. Food & Drug Administration. *Exposure-Response Relationships - Study Design, Data Analysis, and Regulatory Applications.* (2020) on June 3, Available from: https://www.fda.gov/media/71277/download, accessed.

[23] Chatterjee, P, T Anand, KJ Singh, R Rasaily, R Singh, S Das. (2020). Healthcare workers & SARS-CoV-2 Infection in India: A case-control investigation in the time of COVID-19. *Indian J Med Res;* 151: 459-67.

[24] Majumder, M, and KD Mandl. (2020). Early Transmissibility Assessment of a Novel Coronavirus in Wuhan, China. *SSRN Electronic Journal.* https://doi.org/10.2139/ssrn.3524675.

[25] Li, R, W Lu, X Yang, P Feng, O Muqimova, Chen X, and G Wei. (2020). Prediction of the Epidemic of COVID-19 Based on Quarantined Surveillance in China. *MedRxiv.* 2020.02.27.20027169. https://doi.org/10.1101/2020.02.27.20027169.

[26] NCBI, SARS-CoV-2 (Severe acute respiratory syndrome coronavirus 2) *Sequences,* 2020, (https://www.ncbi.nlm.nih.gov/genbank/sars-cov-2-seqs/).

In: Impacts and Implications of COVID-19 ISBN: 978-1-53619-670-2
Editors: Anand Sharma et al.

Chapter 10

COVID-19 Onset: Concussion on Society, Global Environment, and Impediment

Abhishek Sharma*
Department of Business Administration,
Bareilly College, Bareilly, Uttar Pradesh, India

Abstract

The COVID-19 pandemic is considered the most significant worldwide well-being disaster of the century and the best test humankind has looked at since the Second World War. In December 2019, another irresistible respiratory illness rose in Wuhan, Hubei territory, China, and was named by the World Health Organization as COVID-19 (coronavirus malady 2019). Another class of crown infection, known as SARS-CoV-2 (severe intense respiratory disorder coronavirus 2), has been seen as answerable for the event of this ailment. The historical backdrop of human progress is worried. There are cases of extreme disorders brought about by various vi-stratagems as indicated by the World Health Organization

* Corresponding Author's E-mail: sharma.abhishek.01984@gmail.com.

report (WHO as of April 18, 2020). The present flare-up of COVID-19 has influenced more than 2164111 individuals and murdered over 146,198 individuals in more than 200 nations all around the world. Till now, there is no report of any clinically endorsed antiviral medications or immunizations that are successful against COVID-19. It has quickly spread far and wide, presenting gigantic well-being, monetary, environmental, and social difficulties to the whole human populace. The coronavirus flare-up is seriously disturbing the worldwide economy. Practically all the countries are battling to hinder the transmission of the ailment by testing and treating patients, isolating speculated people through contact following, limiting huge social affairs, incomplete lockdown, etc. This paper portrays the effect of COVID-19 on society and the worldwide environment, and the possible manners by which the ailment can be controlled have likewise been discussed that.

Keywords: COVID-19, pandemics, health, transmission, global emergencies

Introduction

Pandemics, by and large, are not simply genuine general well-being concerns; instead, these trigger awful financial and political emergencies in the tainted nations. COVID-19, aside from turning into the best risk to the worldwide general well-being of the century, is being considered a pointer of disparity and deficiency of social headway. As is inferred in the name COVID-19, 'CO' means 'crown,' 'VI' for 'infection,' and 'D' for sickness and 19 speaks to the time of its event. Coronavirus is a solitary abandoned RNA infection with a width extending from 80 to 120 nm. The first present-day COVID-19 pandemic was accounted for in December 2019 in Wuhan, Hubei area, China, and most beginning cases were related to source disease from a fish discount showcase (Huang et al., 2020). From that point forward, the malady quickly circumnavigated the globe and has, in the long run, influenced each mainland except Antarctica. It has been categorized as a pandemic by the World Health Organization (World Health Organization, 2020). Global Committee on Taxonomy of Viruses (ICTV) named the infection as an extreme intense respiratory disorder coronavirus 2 (SARS-CoV-2) [1, 2]. As indicated by WHO, in 2002–2003, more than 8000 individuals endured, and 774 kicked the bucket of a coronavirus called SARS. In 2012, the MERS-CoV pandemic broke out, infecting more than 2494 people and executing more than 858 lives worldwide (WHO, 2004, 2013). Coronaviruses have a place with an enormous assorted group of vi-stratagems. These can be classified into four genera specifically, α-, β-, γ-, and δ. All the recently examined coronaviruses liable for the overall spread of the pandemic; to be specific, SARS, MERS-CoV, and SARS-CoV- 2 are β-coronaviruses. Much AI-based research is conducted to estimate the spread [3, 4] and diagnose the infection [5].

Aside from COVID-19, human development has seen at any rate five pandemics in the present century, for example, H1N1 in 2009, polio in 2014, Ebola (out broke in West Africa in 2014), Zika (2016), and Ebola. Along these lines, COVID-19 flare-up was pronounced as the 6th general well-being crisis of global worry on January 30, 2020, by the WHO. These overall episodes triggered countless fatalities, morbidities and cost billions of dollars. Contrasted with different disorders and their particular weights, COVID-19 will probably cause a lot or more noteworthy human enduring than various infectious illnesses in the entire world. Moreover, other worldwide ecological changes, for example, soil degradation, ozone layer exhaustion, contamination, and urbanization, changing conditions, make an unquestionable danger to our planet and human well-being. A dangerous atmospheric deviation has its underlying foundations in the modern turn of events, with the big arrival of CO_2 during the mechanical insurgency and past, finally permitting the nursery impact to happen. Somewhat COVID-19 episode might be considered as an indirect result of worldwide ecological changes. Other than its upsetting impacts on human life, the novel coronavirus infection (COVID-19) can significantly log jam the economy of China, the USA, or India yet in addition to the world overall. Along these lines, medical services faculty, administrators, and people in general, when all is said in done, need to show solidarity and fight shoulder to shoulder for counteraction and control of the pandemic. Our primary center is to feature the effects of COVID-19 on conditions and society in the current paper. An endeavor has been made to bring up the preventive courses for limiting the hazard factors.

COVID-19: A Global Kind

The flare-up of the new coronavirus disease, COVID-19, was initiated from the Hunan fish showcase in Wuhan city of China in December 2019, and within a few months, it has ended up being a worldwide well-being crisis. Live creatures like bat, frog, snake, flying animal, marmot, and bunny are now and again sold at the Hunan fish advertise [6]. A genomic investigation uncovered that SARS-CoV-2 is phylogenetically identified with a severe, intense respiratory disorder like (SARS-like) bat vi-stratagems. Bats could, in this manner, be the viable essential source. Even though the transitional wellspring of cause and move to people isn't known, the quick human to the human spreading ability of this infection has been set up. According to the most recent update of WHO on April 18, 2020, the episode of COVID-19 had spread to more than 200 nations. Around 146,198 individuals had kicked the bucket in the wake of getting the respiratory infection out of almost 2,164,111 confirmed cases, while in a lot of 402,989 individuals have recuperated from the malady. These numbers are evolving quickly.

In excess of 200 nations/districts have announced confirmed COVID-19 cases, including China, Italy, Iran, S. Korea, India, Switzerland, Taiwan, USA, Sweden, Singapore, Sri Lanka, France, Australia, Malaysia, Spain, United Arab Emirates, UK, Nepal, Finland, Netherlands, Japan, Belgium, Russia, Thailand, Philippines, Cambodia, and Germany. In the wake of hitting China in January 2020, COVID-19 seriously outbroke nations like South Korea, Iran, and Italy in late February and early March 2020. To the extent the quantity of COVID contaminated patients is concerned, the USA is at the highest priority on the rundown, followed by Spain. In the USA, in excess of 30,000 individuals kicked the bucket of this infection. As indicated by the report of the Chinese government and the WHO, the present flare-up has contaminated exactly 84,180 individuals in China, out of which more than 4642 people have kicked the bucket so far as of April 18. The first instance of coronavirus episode in India was accounted for on January 30, 2020, in Kerala's Thrissur area when an understudy had to get back from Wuhan University in China. The Health Ministry of India has confirmed 14,378 instances of coronavirus disease and 480 passings in the nation so far on 18.04.2020. From one perspective, the high transmissibility of the infection is liable for its overall spread. The improvement and availability of universal travel and the travel industry could be an explanation behind its further general spread then again. Consistently, various pieces of the world arrange different strict, socio-social, scientific, sport, and political mass get-together celebrations. These sorts of mass accumulate things are probably going to misrepresent a significant number of the hazard variables of COVID- 19 and have verifiably been related with flare-ups of sickness both in nearby and worldwide levels. The rise and spread of COVID-19 from Asia to the Americas, Africa, and Europe speak to a global dish-demic danger.

COVID-19: Comprehensiveness Haleness

The connection between human well-being and malady is neither another idea nor another subject. The development of COVID-19 in China toward the finish of 2019 has caused an enormous worldwide flare-up and is a significant general medical problem. This infection is profoundly irresistible and can be transmitted through beads and close contact. The human-to-human spreading of the disease happens because of close contact with a contaminated individual presented to hacking, wheezing, respiratory beads, or pressurized canned products. These mist concentrates can infiltrate the human body (respiratory framework) by means of inhalation through the nose or mouth. The clinical range for people with COVID-19 contamination ranges from mellow or non-specific signs and side effects of intense respiratory sickness, for example, fever, hack, weakness, the brevity of breath, to severe pneumonia with respiratory disappointment and septic stun, which are fundamentally the same as different coronavirus maladies. The presenting highlights of COVID-19 sickness in grown-ups are articulated. It involves extraordinary significance to explain the connection between COVID-19 and resistant rheumatologic patients. Thinking about the brisk and wild spread of the plague, the well-being of rheumatic patients involves prime concern. COVID-19 being a respiratory sickness, harm of the tissues of Lungs is very self-evident; however, there is the report that other organs and tissues may likewise be influenced. Since viral shedding in plasma or serum is regular in respiratory tract diseases, there is a chance of transmission of coronaviruses through the transfusion of labile blood items. COVID-19 is a significant general well-being worry for the total populace and is the primary source of hospitalization and passing, particularly for the center and mature age individuals in the influenced nations.

COVID-19 AND AUSTERITY

The connection between human well-being and malady is neither another idea nor another subject. The rise of COVID-19 in China toward the finish of 2019 has caused an enormous worldwide flare-up and is a significant general medical problem. This infection is profoundly irresistible and can be transmitted through beads and close contact. The human-to-human spreading of the disease happens because of close contact with a contaminated individual presented to hacking, wheezing, respiratory beads or mist concentrates. These pressurized canned products can infiltrate the human body (respiratory framework) by means of inhalation through the nose or mouth. The clinical range for people with COVID-19 contamination ranges from gentle or non-specific signs and side effects of intense respiratory sickness, for example, fever, hack, exhaustion, the brevity of breath, to severe pneumonia with respiratory disappointment and septic stun, which are fundamentally the same as different coronavirus ailments. The presenting highlights of COVID-19 malady in grown-ups are articulated. It involves incredible significance to explain the relationship between COVID-19 and safe rheumatologic patients. Contemplating the snappy and berserk spread of the pestilence, the well-being of rheumatic patients involves prime concern. COVID-19 being a respiratory ailment, harm of the tissues of Lungs is very self-evident, yet there is the report that other organs and tissues may likewise be influenced. Since viral shedding in plasma or serum is regular in respiratory tract diseases, there is a chance of transmission of coronaviruses through the transfusion of labile blood items. COVID-19 is a significant general well-being worry for the total populace and is the primary source of hospitalization and passing, particularly for the center and mature age individuals in the influenced nations.

COVID-19 AND GLOBAL AMBIANCE

From the earliest starting point of progress, people, bit by bit, began controlling nature for its own benefit. So as to fulfill the interest of expanding the populace, industrialization and urbanization got unavoidable, and the undeniable significance ended up being detrimental to the worldwide condition. Further, ecological worries include air contamination, water contamination, environmental change, ozone layer consumption, an unnatural weather change, exhaustion of groundwater level, difference in biodiversity and biological system, arsenic tainting, and some more. An Earth-wide temperature boost is a consequence of the expanding grouping of ozone-harming substances (CO_2, CH_4, N_2O, and so forth). Out of the longing to drive nature according to their own impulses and want, people began devastating nature from numerous points of view as an unavoidable outcome condition contamination has become a significant issue of the current day.

Yet, because of the uncommon episode of COVID-19, pretty much every of all shapes and sizes urban areas and towns in the influenced nations like China, Taiwan, Italy, USA, France, Spain, Turkey, Iran, Germany, S Korea, U.K, India, Australia and some more, is under fractional of absolute lockdown for an extensive stretch of time extending from half a month up to a couple of months. All neighborhood and focal organizations worldwide have genuinely put a prohibition on the free development of their residents outside their homes so as to evade community transmission. The different strict, social, social scientific, sport, and political mass get-together occasions like Hajj, Olympics, and so on are dropped. Other sorts of enterprises are not working, a wide range of movements are dropped. Then, endeavors to limit transmission of the SARS-CoV-2 by confining the development have had a remarkable environmental impact. Due to the non-working of enterprises, the modern waste discharge has diminished to a considerable degree. Vehicles are not really found on the streets, coming about right around zero release of greenhouse gases and poisonous modest suspended particles to the earth. Because of lesser interest in intensity in ventures, utilization of petroleum products or traditional vitality sources has been brought down impressively. Biological systems are in effect enormously recouped. In numerous large urban communities, the occupants are encountering an unmistakable sky for the first time in their lives. The contamination level in places of interest, for example, backwoods, ocean, seashores, slope zones, and so on, is likewise contracting to a great extent. The ozone layer has been found to have been resuscitated somewhat. The dish demic has shown its differentiating result on human progress, as in, on the one hand, it has executed overall devastation, yet made an exceptionally positive effect on the world condition then again.

The Global Blueprint for COVID-19 Impediment and Management

COVID-19 is a worldwide risk that requires a worldwide reaction, including all nations. Governments ought to be answerable for giving accurate in-arrangement to help the open face this novel contamination. To diminish the harm associated with COVID-19, general well-being and contamination control activities are promptly essential to confine the worldwide spread of the infection. Some Global methodologies are examined beneath to anticipation and control COVID-19 illness.

Narrow Horde Communal Cases

Forestalling SARS-CoV-2 transmission by confining mass social occasions is a significant target of the general human services framework. COVID-19 is spread from individual to individual through direct contact. In this way, the spread of respiratory illnesses during the mass social affair is a significant general well-being worry with the capability of dispersion of these irresistible dis-facilitates. In view of prior information on MERS and SARS diseases, the WHO, so as to lessen the general danger of transmission of COVID-19, has suggested some prudent steps, for example, staying away from close contact with individuals experiencing intense respiratory ailment, regular hand washing with cleanser and water or hand sanitizer especially after direct contact with wiped out individuals or their condition, keeping up hack behavior, and evading unprotected contact with ranch or wild animals and so on. Govt. of various nations deferred a wide range of strict, social, social, scientific, sport, and political mass get-together occasions in different pieces of the world. Some global affairs, for example, Umrah, Hajj, and the Olympic Games have just been suspended so as to keep away from mass social events. Media and data innovation is giving significant backing to the general public for counteraction and control of the COVID-19 outbreak. Thus, confining mass social affairs could be the essential preventive technique for COVID-19.

AID

The episode of COVID-19 has become a clinical danger to the common populace and human services laborers around the world. Since this is another infection, much information about this novel infection is along these lines not accessible. Up until this point, there are no definite antiviral medicines or immunizations for COVID-19 sickness. Subsequently, it is a dire need of time to develop a protected and stable COVID-19 antibody. Hostiles to viral medications like Chloroquine and Hydroxychloroquine have been seen as compelling against COVID-19 in research facility considerations and in-vivo examinations. An ongoing report by Wang et al. uncovered that remdesivir and chloroquine were profoundly compelling in the control of 2019- nCoV in vitro. Since SARS-CoV-2 is an RNA infection, any antibodies viable against other RNA infections, for example, measles, polio, encephalitis B, and influenza, could be the most promising options. Along these lines, research will keep on assuming a significant job to find new medications or immunizations to forestall and control the COVID-19 diseases.

FORESTATION

As indicated by the World Wildlife Fund, woods spread over 30% of the earth's property surface. The relentless developments in the human populace lead to deforestation for assets, ventures, and land for farming or brushing. Rising average temperature and sea levels and the expanded pace of outrageous climate occasions influence the worldwide land and eco-framework, yet in addition human well-being. Deforestations are additionally connected to various sorts of illness because of the feathered creatures, bat-borne viral flare-ups. COVID-19 is a bat-related pestilence. To forestall this episode, billions of dollars are being spent to create analytic, treatment, and medication. Be that as it may, we are ignoring the essential devices of counteraction, for example, forestation and respecting untamed life living spaces. It is along these lines particularly significant for the world to understand the significance of the timberlands and to support afforestation however much as could reasonably be expected all through the world.

CONTROLLING HUMAN POPULACE DEVELOPMENT

Condition change is probably going to affect human well-being. Condition change has been decidedly identified with human influences. A significant factor is fast human populace development, which has been joined by the colossal monetary turn of events and expanding wellsprings of contamination, for example, vehicles and dirtying businesses. In China, the relentless increment in human populace development has led to deforestation, and the individuals eat various sorts of bats, frogs, snakes, feathered creatures, and creatures. COVID-19 is accounted for as a bat-related pandemic that began in China [7].

Uncovering exceedingly helpless populaces to new Pathogens by expanded human migration to recently secluded territories may unite irresistible illnesses. Control of populace development is consequently fundamental in such a manner.

Worldwide Prohibition on Natural Life Exchange

The beginning stage of the COVID-19 flare-up was the Hunan fish showcase, Wuhan, China. China has briefly put a restriction on untamed life markets where creatures, for example, civet, bat, little wolf guy, pangolin, and so forth, are kept alive in little pens while discounted. 60% of developing transferable maladies originate from creatures, and 70% of these should start in wild animals. In this way, the unlimited natural life exchange may improve the dangers of developing new infections. Numerous researchers have encouraged various nations to for all time boycott untamed life markets and businesses. These activities would assist with shielding human lives from future pandemics like COVID-19.

Conclusion

Condition change is one of the most significant and most indispensable difficulties of the 21st century. Disregarding the entirety of their endeavors to reestablish nature during the most recent couple of decades, people could push a couple of strides ahead. In any case, during the most recent couple of months, results of the pandemic have effectively recouped the earth to a considerable degree that should definitely set a positive effect on worldwide environmental change. Whatever be the reason or starting point, the event of COVID-19 has underlined to im-demonstrate the commonly full of feeling association among people and nature. Now of time, it is irreplaceable to control the wellspring of illness, remove the transmission way, and utilize the current medications and intend to control the advancement of the ailment proactively. Like all the first disasters on the earth, let all be hopeful enough that individuals will definitely prevail upon the pandemic at the appointed time of time, however they should know the cutoff points to which they can push nature before it is past the point of no return.

References

[1] Gorbalenya, A. E., Baker, S. C., Baric, R. S., de Groot, R. J., Drosten, C., Gulyaeva, A. A., et al., (2020). Severe acute respiratory syndrome-related coronavirus: the species and its viruses - a statement of the Coronavirus Study Group. *Bio Rxiv.*

[2] Backer, J. A., Klinkenberg, D., & Wallinga, J. (2020). Incubation period of 2019 novel coronavirus (2019-nCoV) infections among travelers from Wuhan, China, 20-28 January 2020. *Euro surveillance: bulletin Europeen sur les maladies transmissibles = European communicable disease bulletin*, *25*(5), 2000062.

[3] Agrawal, A., Arora, R., Arora, R., Agrawal, P., (2021). Applications of Artificial Intelligence and Internet of Things for Detection and Future Directions to Fight against COVID-19. In the edited book on *Emerging Technologies for Battling Covid-19*, 107-119, Springer.

[4] Madaan, A., Roy, A., Gupta, C., Agrawal, P., Sharma, A., Bologa, C., Prodan, R., (2021). XCOVNet: Chest X-ray Image Classification for COVID-19 Early Detection Using Convolutional Neural Networks. *New Generation Computing*, 1-15.

[5] Agrawal, P., Madaan, V., Roy, A., Kumari, R., Deore, Harshal, (2021). FOCOMO: Forecasting and monitoring the worldwide spread of COVID-19 using machine learning methods, *Journal of Interdisciplinary Mathematics,* 1-25.

[6] Huang, C., Wang, Y., Li, X., Ren, L., Zhao, J., Hu, Y., et al., (2020). Clinical features of patients infected with 2019 novel coronavirus in Wuhan, China. *Lancet* 395, 497–506.

[7] Fan, Y., Zhao, K., Shi, Z. L., et al., 2019. Bat coronaviruses in China. *Viruses* 11, 210.

EDITORS' CONTACT INFORMATION

Anand Sharma
Assistant Professor,
Department of Computer Science and Engineering,
Mody University of Science and Technology,
Lakshmangarh, Rajasthan, India
anand.glee@gmail.com

Prateek Agrawal
Post Doctoral Researcher,
Institute of Information Technology,
University of Klagenfurt, Austria
Associate Professor and HOD- Intelligent Systems
Discipline of Computer Science & Engineering
Lovely Professional University,
Punjab, India

Vishu Madaan
Assistant Professor,
School of Computer Science Engineering,
Lovely Professional University, India

Anuj Agarwal
COO, Taifa Gas Tanzania Ltd., Tanzania

INDEX

A

B

C

D

E

F

G

H

I

J

L

U

V

W